CASE STUDIES IN BREAST CANCER

CASE STUDIES IN BREAST CANCER

Adrian Harnett
M.B. B.S., MRCP, FRCR

Consultant in Clinical Oncology
Beatson Oncology Centre
Western Infirmary
Glasgow, UK

GMM

LONDON ● SAN FRANCISCO

GMM

© 2002
Greenwich Medical Media Limited
137 Euston Road
London
NW1 2AA

870 Market Street, Ste 720
San Francisco
CA 94109, USA

ISBN 1 84110 000 5

First published 2002

Visit our website at:
www.greenwich-medical.co.uk

Distributed worldwide by Plymbridge Distributors Ltd and in the USA by Jamco Distribution

Typeset by Phoenix Photosetting, Chatham, Kent
Printed in Great Britain by The Bath Press

Contents

Foreword

The diagnosis of breast cancer is often devastating. The patient is usually very well and has no inkling that they have cancer, apart from perhaps the recent onset of a lump in the breast. On the other hand, they are usually aware of the seriousness of the disease and the underlying connotations. They may well have dependent family members.

Therefore, it is all the more important that they are treated sensitively and by a team with considerable experience in the combined management of this illness.

This book is a series of case histories of patients treated almost exclusively in the Breast Unit and Beatson Oncology Centre at the Western Infirmary, Glasgow by the multidisciplinary team. Adrian Harnett joined the unit over 13 years ago and is involved in every aspect of their care. He attends the preoperative ward rounds every week and gives valuable oncological input at the time of primary surgical management.

I recommend and encourage you to read this book, which illustrates just a few of the many challenges that have confronted us over the years.

Professor W D George
Regius Professor of Surgery
University of Glasgow
July 2001

Preface

When I first was a trainee in the Department of Radiotherapy at St Bartholomew's Hospital I was fortunate enough to be taught by Professor Arthur Jones. For every case, he would ask "What is the catch?" As a result, even in what may appear straightforward cases, I always looked for the potential problem or difficulty. It has become intuitive in my routine care of patients.

The following cases illustrate the diverse management of the very common condition of breast cancer but they all have 'catches' ranging from diagnostic dilemmas to management problems. Cases are sequenced through the book starting with diagnosis, early stage disease through to locally advanced disease, localised (single site) metastatic disease and widespread metastatic disease, including palliative care. All cases are real patients who have come under my care, either at initial presentation or for advice concerning their further management. Very little information in the text has been altered and when this has occurred it is for reasons such as patient request. Some management decisions are controversial and some cases were initially treated many years ago, so their earlier management would be very different now. A few patients have only recently been referred to me, having been managed previously by another clinician. Also, many patients are ongoing in their care and this may give the impression that the case history is incomplete – correctly so!

By and large, the text for the illustrations has been kept very brief and often it does not describe the abnormalities in the photographs. This is to enable you to decide what the abnormality, or abnormalities are and, so you are not given answers prematurely. Usually they are described later in the text. Questions are provided throughout the text and illustrations placed, where possible, so that answers follow later. You may wish to look at the illustrations first before reading the accompany text.

Breast cancer is a very challenging disease to treat and I hope the case descriptions of patients' treated in the centre illustrate the complexity of management, give you new ideas and encourage us all to improve the multi-disciplinary management of breast cancer.

July 2001
Adrian Harnett

Acknowledgements

There are many people to whom I express thanks for their advice and encouragement in making the completion of this book possible. By naming them I am bound to leave out some important contributions so firstly I would like to thank all my clinical colleagues and the multidisciplinary team involving Breast Surgeons, Pharmacists, Breast Care Nurses and Clinical and Ward Nurses, secretarial and medical illustration staff.

I particularly express my thanks to my surgical colleagues Professor David George, Mr Arnie Purushotham, Miss Julie Doughty, Mr Chris Simpson and Mr Chris Morran. I value the input of Pathologists Drs Liz Mallon and Iain Graham, Radiologist Dr Nigel McMillan and Palliative Care Physicians Professor John Welsh and Dr Kirsty Muirhead. The assistance of Sharon Napier, Caroline Eadie and Sharon Sutherland in Medical Illustration at the Western Infirmary was invaluable as was the assistance of Geoff Nuttall and Gavin Smith from Greenwich Medical Media and Nora Naughton. Ailsa Macleod gave me secretarial support.

AstraZeneca made the project possible and so I would particularly thank them and Julie Lardelli. I am grateful for the patience and encouragement of my wife Sally and the enthusiasm of Lynne Arrol.

Finally, this book is the story of an illness borne bravely by many patients and described in the following pages. They are the biggest contributors of all and it has been my privilege to be involved in their care. I thank them for all they have taught me.

Case 1: Breast conservation or mastectomy?

Look at the photograph (Fig 1.1). Which breast has been treated for breast cancer?

There are different factors, which may influence a decision about whether to perform breast conservation surgery or mastectomy. Sometimes mastectomy is indicated on several grounds; sometimes there may be just one overriding factor. These may include:

- Size of the primary
- Location
- Size of the breast
- Multifocal tumours and extensive DCIS
- Patient desire (which may be mastectomy when conservation could be performed or vice versa)
- Age of the patient (in general older patients are more willing to have mastectomy, younger patients breast conservation surgery).

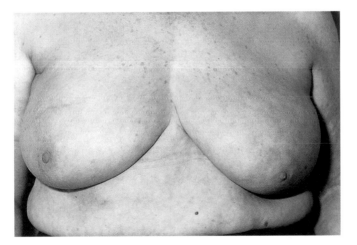

Figure 1.1 Breast after conservation surgery and radiotherapy.

A 70-year-old patient noticed a lump in the inferior aspect of the left breast below the nipple. Clinically she had a 2.5 cm tumour, which was confirmed on FNA and trucut biopsies although the mammogram was unremarkable. She underwent breast conservation surgery but had no axillary surgery. Histology confirmed a 2 cm grade II invasive ductal carcinoma that was completely excised.

The tumour was strongly receptor positive and she was commenced on adjuvant tamoxifen. She received a course of postoperative radiotherapy to the left breast and gland areas using a standard 4 field megavoltage isocentric technique. She tolerated this treatment well.

At a routine follow-up with mammography, an abnormality was detected in the right breast suspicious of malignancy. Localisation of the lesion was carried out and confirmed malignancy. In spite of her age and her previous experience of breast cancer, she wished again to have breast conservation surgery, which was carried out. Histology revealed a 5 mm grade I invasive ductal carcinoma that was excised with clear margins and did not involve any of the 19 lymph nodes. The tumour was strongly receptor positive.

Her hormonal treatment was changed from tamoxifen to megestrol acetate and she received a course of postoperative radiotherapy to the right breast alone. She remained on this hormonal treatment for five years.

She remains well and disease-free 12 years after the initial diagnosis of breast cancer. She is extremely pleased by the cosmetic result obtained from bilateral breast conservation surgery and irradiation. For the left-sided tumour this included the supraclavicular fossa and axilla as well as the breast, because no axillary surgery had been performed. However, current policy is always to carry out surgical staging of the axilla by axillary clearance or sampling or possibly sentinal node biopsy.

Case 2: The influence of coexisting disease

A 40-year-old premenopausal patient presented with recent onset of a lump in the right breast. Clinically, it had the characteristics of a carcinoma and this was confirmed on biopsy. She had a past medical history of Crohn's disease. Wide local excision and axillary dissection were carried out for an 18 mm grade 2 invasive ductal carcinoma. The tumour was 80% oestrogen receptor positive and did not involve any of the 15 lymph nodes.

What adjuvant therapy would you plan for this patient?

As she had breast conservation surgery she received a routine course of postoperative radiotherapy to the right breast alone receiving a standard fractionation followed by a boost to the site of local excision. This treatment was well tolerated.

As the tumour was strongly receptor positive it would be appropriate to give hormonal treatment. She was commenced on adjuvant tamoxifen 20 mg a day and should continue this treatment for five years. Combination hormonal treatment is being increasingly employed as studies have been carried out in both the adjuvant and advanced setting (including the UKCCCR adjuvant breast cancer (ABC) premenopausal trial, trials of tamoxifen and LHRH agonists in advanced breast cancer, the CRC trial with an LHRH agonist and tamoxifen and the ATAC trial in postmenopausal patients in patients with early breast cancer). Therefore ovarian suppression could be considered as adjuvant treatment in this patient. However, ovarian suppression by radiation menopause or surgical oophrectomy are best avoided in the presence of Crohn's disease. It could be achieved using a LHRH analogue goserelin (Zoladex) if it was felt necessary and indicated to achieve ovarian suppression.

Similarly chemotherapy with, for example, cyclophosphamide methotrexate and 5 fluorouracil is less well tolerated in the presence of Crohn's disease, causing more GI upset. In this case it was not felt necessary to give chemotherapy.

Case 3: The difficult diagnosis

A 47-year-old office worker presented with a discharge from her right nipple and later the right breast became painful and swollen. Clinical examination revealed erythema of the breast and discharge from the nipple, which on cytological examination revealed suspicious cells. Mammography revealed a 8 cm lesion in the right breast; fine needle aspiration from the large poorly defined mass in the breast did not reveal malignant cells.

Discuss the differential diagnosis and management

It was thought the patient could have an inflammatory breast carcinoma or possibly a phylloides tumour on mammographic appearances. She could also have a breast abscess.

A trucut and then open biopsy were performed and neither showed any evidence of malignancy. She was treated with a course of antibiotics and the signs of inflammation and swelling of the breast largely resolved. However, two months later she had a recurrence and again was treated with a further course of antibiotics. Again she had a response but the swelling, (Figures 3.1 and 3.2) erythema and oedema of the breast recurred.

What management would you recommend?

Further cytology and biopsy were performed which now confirmed malignancy with a poorly differentiated ductal carcinoma (Figures 3.3, 3.4 and 3.5). Staging investigations were all clear.

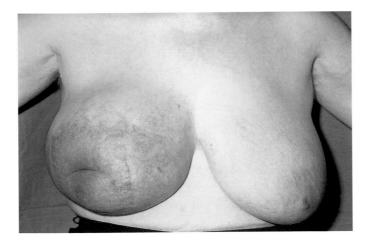

Figure 3.1.

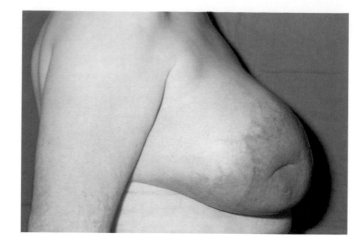

Figures 3.1 and 3.2 Inflammation of the right breast. Note central scar from open biopsy.

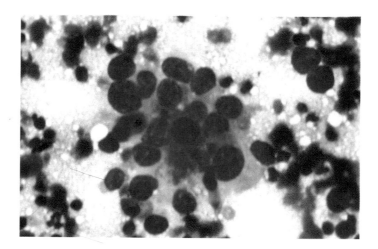

Figure 3.3 Cytology showed malignant cells.

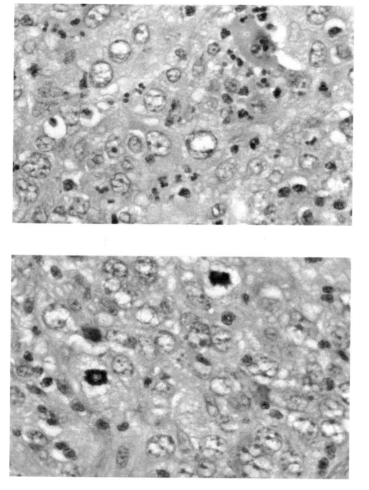

Figures 3.4 and 3.5 Invasive breast cancer with pleomorphic cells (3.4) and mitotic figures (3.5).

What treatment would you recommend?

She received neoadjuvant chemotherapy with 5 fluorouracil, adriamycin and cyclophosphamide. She received six courses of treatment with an excellent response. There was good resolution of the oedema, erythema and regression of the poorly defined mass. A mastectomy and axillary dissection were then carried out. Histology revealed no residual invasive tumour but there were changes consistent with her response to chemotherapy. There was no involvement of the 14 lymph nodes examined.

In view of the fact that she had a poorly differentiated inflammatory carcinoma with large groups and sheets of pleomorphic cells, she was given a course of postoperative chest wall irradiation over four weeks.

Over five years later she remains well and disease free.

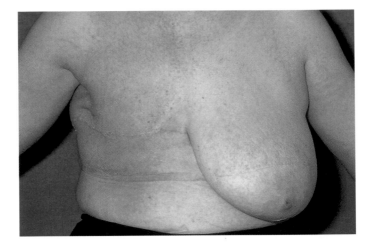

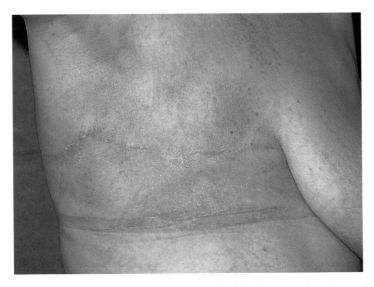

Figures 3.6 and 3.7   Right mastectomy and slight skin pigmentation due to chest wall irradiation.

Comment

The diagnosis of inflammatory breast cancer and breast abscess or mastitis can be difficult to differentiate. This patient illustrates original negative tests for malignancy despite even an open biopsy. It would appear that the inflammatory carcinoma had an element of sepsis and mastitis which made diagnosis more difficult.

These tumours are aggressive and difficult to control locally, especially when primary treatment is mastectomy, (which used to be the standard management). When chemotherapy is given neoadjuvantly, long term control and possibly cure can be obtained, as illustrated in this case.

Case 4: Sequential bilateral breast carcinoma

A 48-year-old journalist presented with a lump in the left breast and, following confirmation of the diagnosis, underwent a mastectomy and axillary dissection for a small grade 2 invasive ductal carcinoma that was node negative and strongly receptor positive. She was treated with adjuvant tamoxifen alone and two years later underwent left breast reconstruction. Her periods stopped when she was commenced on tamoxifen. There was no family history of breast disease.

Six years later and while she was still on tamoxifen she developed a lump in the right breast. FNA revealed malignant cells and mammography supported the diagnosis of malignancy. Right wide local excision and axillary clearance were performed for a 6 mm grade 3 invasive ductal carcinoma that was 100% oestrogen receptor positive. One of 15 lymph nodes was involved.

What further treatment would you recommend?

This postmenopausal patient had developed a contralateral breast carcinoma whilst being on adjuvant tamoxifen which she had not wished to discontinue after five years. As the second tumour was strongly receptor positive she was changed to anastrozole (arimidex) which is a third generation aromatase inhibitor. As she was only just post-menopausal, had a high grade tumour with axillary node involvement and had developed the tumour whilst on hormonal treatment, she was offered adjuvant chemotherapy and was given six courses of cyclophosphamide, methotrexate and 5 fluorouracil. (An anthracycline combination would probably be used now in preference to CMF.) She would have been ineligible for any trial of combined chemoendocrine therapy as she had had a previous malignancy. As breast conservation had been performed, she received a course of postoperative radiotherapy to the right breast in the standard fashion with a boost to the site of local excision on completion of whole breast radiotherapy.

Case 5: Genetic disease/ Cancer family syndrome

A 52-year-old postmenopausal patient presented with a lump in the upper outer quadrant of the right breast. She had a hysterectomy with preservation of one ovary at the age of 37. She had been on HRT for five years and this had just been discontinued. She has three daughters. Sixteen years ago she had a right hemicolectomy for polyposis coli. Two of her brothers died of carcinoma of the colon.

FNA of the lump in the breast did not reveal any evidence of malignancy and bilateral mammography was normal. However, trucut biopsy revealed infiltrating carcinoma.

She was admitted and wide local excision and axillary dissection carried out. During her inpatient stay she developed haematuria and an IVP suggested a primary tumour of the kidney (Figure 5.1). CT scan confirmed a renal mass (Figures 5.2 and 5.3). A left nephrectomy and removal of the ureter was performed and histology revealed a papillary transitional cell carcinoma arising from the renal pelvis. Excision appeared complete. Pathology of the breast revealed a 15 mm grade 2 invasive ductal carcinoma. It was completely excised and 100% oestrogen receptor positive. There was no involvement of the axillary nodes.

What further treatment would you recommend?

What advice would you give concerning screening of other family members?

She was commenced on tamoxifen and received a course of postoperative radiotherapy in the routine fashion to the right breast following breast conservation surgery. The transitional cell carcinoma of the renal pelvis is a slightly unusual tumour but was completely excised. She does not require any further treatment for this malignancy. However, she does require regular review of the renal tract to ensure she has not developed a transitional cell carcinoma on the right side or in the bladder.

Her daughters, the eldest of whom is 34, are being regularly screened already for colorectal cancer. They should be referred to the high risk clinic for yearly breast examinations probably from age 35 and biennial mammography. The patient and family could be referred to the genetics unit for counselling, plotting of the family tree and assessing the risk of genetic disease. Testing for BRCA1 and BRCA2 would be considered and discussed. A further complication is that one of her daughters is already employed in the genetics unit.

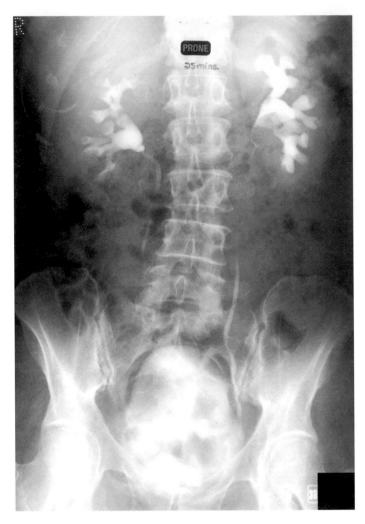

Figure 5.1 Intravenous urogram taken 25 minutes after injection of contrast.

Just prior to completion of five years of tamoxifen, routine follow-up mammography showed an abnormality in the left breast which had the appearance of DCIS. Needle localisation biopsy and wide local excision were carried out and the final pathology revealed an area of DCIS extending over an area of at least 17 mm. The excision margins were clear by at least 9 mm. The cavity shavings were free from tumour. The DCIS was of comedo type, nuclear grade 3 with necrosis. There was a 2.8 mm focus of grade 2 ductal carcinoma which was oestrogen receptor negative.

What further management would you propose?

Further surgery should be considered with a view to axillary staging. However, it was felt that as there was such a small focus of invasive disease

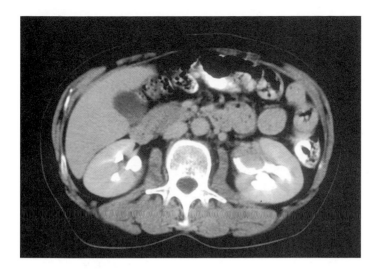

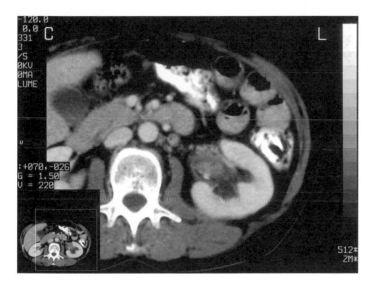

Figures 5.2 and 5.3   CT cuts at the renal levels.

it would be extremely unlikely for there to be any axillary node involvement. Axillary surgery was therefore not performed. However, she received a course of postoperative radiotherapy to the left breast, boosting the site of local excision. Since the tumour and DCIS occurred whilst being on tamoxifen it was discontinued. As the tumour was oestrogen receptor negative she was not given second line hormone treatment. Finally, it was considered that chemotherapy was not necessary or appropriate.

Further comment

When discussing the management of transitional cell carcinoma in bladder, it transpired that the patient smokes 15 cigarettes a day. Transitional cell carcinoma of the urinary tract is linked with smoking and she therefore should be advised to discontinue. However, she has contracted the disease at a fairly young age and it may be more likely that she has a genetic predisposition.

Case 6: HRT and other hormonal issues

A 54-year-old housewife sought medical advice having noticed a lump in her right breast in the upper outer quadrant. She felt well and had no other symptoms. She had had a hysterectomy and bilateral salpingo-oophrectomy four years ago for menorrhagia and she had been on hormone replacement therapy (HRT) ever since. She had two adopted children and had no family history of breast disease. FNA revealed malignant cells. Mammography had been performed three years previously and had been normal. Recent mammogram showed appearances consistent with malignancy. Following confirmation of the diagnosis of breast carcinoma, wide local excision and axillary clearance were carried out. She made a good post operative recovery.

Histology reported a 9 mm grade 2 invasive ductal carcinoma that was 40% oestrogen receptor positive and did not involve any of the 17 lymph nodes removed.

What adjuvant therapy would you recommend?

What advice would you give regarding HRT?

In summary, this postmenopausal patient has had breast conservation surgery for a very small symptomatic rather than screen detected tumour that was receptor positive and node negative. It would be standard treatment to give her a course of postoperative radiotherapy to the right breast alone using paired glancing megavoltage fields. She received 46 Gy in 23 fractions followed by a boost to the site of local excision of a further 12 Gy in 4 fractions using 9 MEV electrons. It would also be appropriate to give her tamoxifen for five years. However, there is uncertainty about the benefit of tamoxifen beyond five years. She could be considered then for entry into one of the adjuvant hormone trials of treatment duration, such as randomising after 5 years of tamoxifen to continue or not (the ATTOM trial). The low risk of endometrial carcinoma with longer duration of tamoxifen is irrelevant as she had a hysterectomy. She in fact was entered into the ATAC study looking at anastrozole or tamoxifen alone or in combination.

The question of HRT is not clear. With the lack of data concerning the use of HRT in patients who have previously had breast cancer the advice usually is given to stop this therapy. There is concern that it may provoke or promote recurrent breast cancer but, if this is the case, the risk is small. Unfortunately, on stopping HRT, the patients may develop quite severe menopausal symptoms and this may be exacerbated by hormonal treatment such as tamoxifen. Within the ATAC trial, HRT therapy has to be discontinued.

The patient remains well and disease free two years following entry into the ATAC trial.

Case 7: Adoption after breast cancer

A 41-year-old accountant had noticed a lump in the left breast in the upper outer quadrant. It had been present for a few weeks and measured 3.5 cm. FNA was malignant. She initially thought she was pregnant so mammography was slightly delayed. It showed five separate lesions in the left breast. A left mastectomy and axillary clearance was performed for five separate invasive grade 3 ductal carcinomas. The largest measured 27 mm in diameter. There was lymphatic invasion in the breast and involvement of one of 28 lymph nodes removed. The tumours were all receptor negative.

There was no family history of breast cancer.

She was extremely concerned about her fertility. Her only child aged two and a half had been conceived by artificial insemination using her husband's sperm. She had many questions about her future fertility, IVF, artificial insemination and adoption.

What management would you recommend?

This is a premenopausal patient who has multifocal high grade disease that was axillary node positive (1 node) and receptor negative. She must be at risk of developing metastatic disease and should receive adjuvant chemotherapy. She was entered into an adjuvant chemotherapy trial (the Scottish epirubicin CMF or NEAT trial) and drew the anthracycline arm. She therefore received four courses of epirubicin followed by four courses of CMF chemotherapy. At completion of chemotherapy she was given postoperative radiotherapy to the left chest wall and skin flaps as she had multifocal high grade node positive disease and was felt to be at risk of local recurrence. Staging investigations performed before starting chemotherapy were carried out, as she had five tumours, but did not show any evidence of metastatic disease.

Her periods returned three months after completing chemotherapy. It is difficult to give advice concerning family planning after treatment for multifocal high grade disease. Her fertility would be adversely affected by chemotherapy even although her periods had returned initially. It would be wise to caution the patient from becoming pregnant within the next few years but time moves on and she is not going to be so fertile at the age of 45. She may also have difficulty anyway in conceiving with the previous medical history.

In view of this situation she approached adoption and fostering agencies but again they are unlikely to look at the patient's situation favourably. The patient and family will require very careful counselling and support.

Case 8: Breast cancer in pregnancy

A 32-year-old patient presented with a two-month history of swelling of the left breast and some associated discomfort. She initially put the symptom down to having stopped breastfeeding and subsequently immediately got pregnant. At a routine antenatal clinic she sought advice due to the discomfort in her left breast. She had three children and was 14 weeks pregnant. There was no family history of breast disease.

Clinical examination revealed a diffuse mass in the left breast with associated erythema of the skin. There was mobile left axillary lymphadenopathy. Fine needle aspiration and trucut biopsy of the left breast confirmed invasive breast cancer (Figure 8.1).

What management would you recommend?

Figure 8.1   Trucut biopsy showing invasive carcinoma with lymphatic invasion H&E stain (×400).

The pregnancy was not planned but the patient and her husband wanted to proceed with the pregnancy if possible. She had a rapidly growing breast cancer with history and appearances of classical inflammatory breast carcinoma.

Clinical examination and limited staging investigation (full blood count, biochemistry profile and liver ultrasound) did not reveal any evidence of distant metastases. It was therefore recommended that the pregnancy was terminated and this was carried out prior to further treatment. Chest X-ray and bone scan were also normal.

After termination of pregnancy there was some regression of the left breast mass and axillary lymphadenopathy. She was commenced on chemotherapy with 5 fluorouracil, epirubicin and cyclophosphamide and at the third course of treatment she had a complete clinical remission of the diffuse changes of the left breast, originally over 7 × 8 cm, and the marked lymphadenopathy. She proceeded to a total of six courses of chemotherapy.

What further management would you recommend?

As she presented with an inflammatory breast carcinoma involving the whole breast, and although she had a complete response to treatment, it was decided to perform a mastectomy and axillary clearance. Pathological examination did not reveal any residual invasive disease but there was scattered in situ carcinoma in the breast (Figures 8.2, 8.3 and

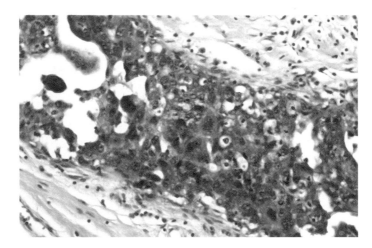

Figure 8.2 Residual in-situ disease only after chemotherapy. Low power magnification (×200).

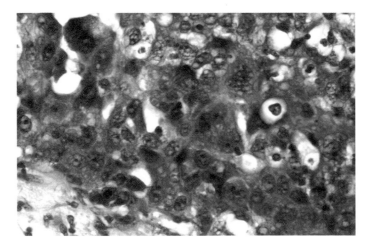

Figures 8.3 High power magnification (×400).

8.4). There was no involvement of the axillary nodes although four nodes showed scarring inferring previous tumour involvement and a good response to chemotherapy (Figure 8.5). The in situ disease was oestrogen receptor negative.

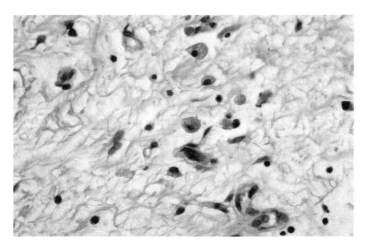

Figures 8.4 Fibrous response and macrophages in breast tissue, no malignant cells seen.

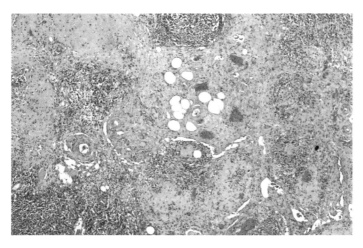

Figures 8.5 Fibrous response (pink staining) indicative of previous tumour in the lymph node.

Discussion

Interpretation of the course of events would be that the inflammatory invasive breast cancer was hormone sensitive and rapidly progressive due to pregnancy. Therefore termination of pregnancy caused regression of her tumour even prior to commencing chemotherapy. The addition of chemotherapy achieved complete regression of her tumour. However, as she had an inflammatory carcinoma there would be a very high risk of local recurrence without definite surgery. Local excision could not be performed as the tumour had involved the whole breast. Therefore mastectomy and axillary clearance were carried out which confirmed an excellent response with no residual invasive tumour.

What further management would you recommend?

Usually postoperative radiotherapy is given following mastectomy for inflammatory breast carcinoma. As there was no residual invasive tumour, it would possibly be reasonable to omit postoperative radiotherapy to the mastectomy scar and chest wall skin flaps. However the patient wanted this additional treatment to try and avoid local recurrence and she received standard radiotherapy treatment over four weeks.

It would be reasonable to give her adjuvant tamoxifen as the original tumour was highly likely to be receptor positive although the DCIS was receptor negative. At present the patient is on no adjuvant treatment. She completed treatment two years ago and remains well and disease free.

Case 9: The doctor patient

A 32-year-old doctor, married to another doctor, presented with a lump in the upper outer quadrant of the right breast which had been present for some time. She had been breast feeding her 10-month-old child and had just weaned the child but the lump persisted. On confirmation of the diagnosis, wide local excision and axillary dissection were carried out for a multifocal invasive lobular carcinoma. The tumours were weakly oestrogen receptor positive. In view of the multifocality of the disease, a right mastectomy was performed. There was also in situ lobular carcinoma. Four of the 19 lymph nodes were involved.

She had three children aged five, three and 10 months. The only relative with breast cancer was her grandmother – this occurred at the age of 74. There was no past medical history of note.

What management would you recommend?

The patient wants advice on contraception. She doesn't want her husband to have a vasectomy and he is not keen for her to have a sterilisation.

How would you advise the patient and her husband?

She was treated with adjuvant chemotherapy receiving two courses of single agent anthracycline. This was poorly tolerated especially with respect to nausea and vomiting despite anti-emetic therapy. After two courses she was changed to CMF chemotherapy and completed six courses of this regimen. Her periods became irregular after chemotherapy but did not stop. She was commenced on tamoxifen and she still continued to menstruate. It is unlikely that ovarian suppression either by radiation, surgery or medically induced would be of additional benefit as her tumour was weakly receptor positive and she was already on one hormonal treatment. However this would have resolved her problem ensuring that she did not get pregnant. As already stated, her husband did not want her to be sterilised. Indeed, she felt she had been through enough treatment and did not want a further operation. She did not want her husband to have a vasectomy in case she died of breast cancer and he wanted to start another family. She was advised to take non-hormonal contraceptive measures such as a condom, cap or IUCD.

Further comment

The patient was not treated with a course of postoperative radiotherapy to the chest wall and supraclavicular fossa. However, with four nodes involved, most centres would now routinely give postoperative radiotherapy to these regions.

Case 10: The high-risk patient

A 37-year-old professional musician initially presented with a lump in the right breast three years ago in Vienna, when she was living in Austria. Further investigation including mammography did not reveal any evidence of malignancy. However, one year later, when she had moved to the UK, the lump in the right breast was larger and a mass developed in the left breast. Apparently, the patient refused FNA and biopsy because she wanted to conceive and breastfeed. Almost nine months later, the patient had a 4 × 5 cm diffuse mass in the left breast with nipple retraction. Core biopsy was positive for invasive carcinoma. Similarly, there was a suspicious mass in the right breast in the upper outer quadrant and core biopsies were positive.

The patient has a five-year-old son from a previous marriage. Her mother and her mother's sister have both had breast cancer, her mother having been treated four years earlier.

Bilateral mastectomy, axillary dissections and immediate breast reconstruction with Becker implants were carried out. Histology from the left breast revealed a 50 mm grade III invasive ductal carcinoma with 19 of 19 lymph nodes involved and the tumour was 100% receptor positive. On the right side there was at least a 50 mm diffuse tumour which was a grade II invasive ductal carcinoma with associated DCIS. Two of 21 lymph nodes were involved and the tumour was again 100% ER positive.

This young women is very concerned about her appearance and her occupation as a professional musician. She is very keen to have another child following her recent marriage.

What advice would you give and what treatment would you recommend?

This patient presents the clinician with considerable challenges and, needless to say, it is a very difficult situation. Her concern with her appearance, desire for a further pregnancy and to breast feed have resulted in a delay in diagnosis and large bilateral tumours. This has been exacerbated by the fact that she has moved three times within the last two years. Her husband works away from home for several months of the year. An appropriate option would have been to treat her with neo-adjuvant chemotherapy. However, as the patient had previous difficulty in accepting surgical management, it was decided to take this opportunity to perform bilateral mastectomy which would probably be better accepted by the patient rather than waiting for response to chemotherapy prior to performing definitive surgery.

However, she is at a considerable risk of metastatic disease and so staging investigations were performed. Bone scan showed increased activity at the right eleventh and the left ninth ribs and the left acetabulum and these would have to be regarded as suspicious of metastatic disease (Figure 10.1).

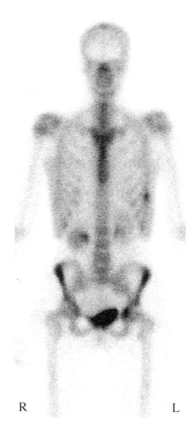

R   L

Figure 10.1   Bone scan appearances at time of staging postoperatively.

Plain radiology was normal and MRI scan of the pelvis was therefore carried out and showed no abnormality of the left acetabulum. It was decided to take an aggressive treatment approach as it had not been possible to prove metastatic disease. The patient was told that it was not practical to think about further pregnancy in view of the diagnosis and the high risk of metastatic disease. Postoperatively gradual inflation of the breast prosthesis was performed. She was entered into the Anglo Celtic study and drew the high dose arm (this study is now closed). She received four courses of adriamycin followed by high dose chemotherapy which was the treatment arm she drew in the study. She had cyclophosphamide, which produced an haemorrhagic cystitis, and then stem cell harvesting. She then received Thiotepa intravenously for four days followed by melphalan on the final day.

She was given routine Mesna. Prior to undergoing this treatment she was seen on several occasions by the clinical psychologist. As both tumours were receptor positive she was commenced on tamoxifen. On completion and recovery from high dose chemotherapy she received a course of radiotherapy to both reconstructed breasts using 50 Gy given by parallel paired megavoltage radiation fields. It was decided not to treat the nodal areas, in particular the left supraclavicular fossa, due to the large volume of tissue already being irradiated and the likelihood of added toxicity. It was also felt that such treatment was unlikely to influence the outcome. The axillae were not irradiated as clearances had been carried out.

The patient remains well several months after completion of therapy although she has slight lymphoedema of the right arm. She is hoping that ovarian function will recover but hormonal analysis (LH, FSH, and serum oestradiol) indicates ovarian failure.

Case 11: The unfit patient

A 69-year-old presented with a neglected carcinoma of the left breast. The tumour had ulcerated through the skin. She was not in any pain.
She had a very complicated past medical history including severe rheumatoid arthritis and seven years ago had an operation on her spine. Now her mobility was limited and she used a zimmer frame. Hypertension had been diagnosed following a CVA and she had since had a further stroke. She also had angina and bronchitis but continued to smoke 15 cigarettes a day.

What line of management would you recommend?

Limited staging investigations were carried out. Liver function tests were normal and chest X-ray did not show any evidence of metastatic pulmonary disease. A bone scan was not arranged and would have been difficult to interpret with respect to metastatic disease due to the severe arthritis. Due to her complicated medical history and the fact she had a locally advanced tumour she was initially commenced on tamoxifen but her tumour progressed. The tumour was not fixed to the chest wall, was technically operable and she was fit enough for anaesthetic. Therefore left mastectomy and axillary dissection were carried out. Histology revealed a 14 mm grade 3 invasive ductal carcinoma with involvement of two of 19 axillary nodes. The tumour was oestrogen receptor negative, which was not surprising as she failed to respond to tamoxifen.

What further management would you recommend?

The patient had poor prognostic disease and was at high risk of developing metastatic disease if she had not done so already. Chemotherapy would usually be standard adjuvant treatment in this setting but the patient was very unfit and likely to develop marked toxicity from this treatment. It therefore was not given. She was at high risk of local recurrence since she had a T4 high grade tumour. She was therefore given a course of postoperative radiotherapy to the left mastectomy scar and chest wall skin flaps. The lymph node areas and particularly the supraclavicular fossa were not included due to co-existing lung disease. Radiotherapy to the supraclavicular fossa would have involved treating the apex of the lung and a considerable lung volume.

Case 12: Pregnancy after cancer/ Neoadjuvant chemotherapy

A 33-year-old sales assistant presented with a lump in the right breast. It rapidly increased in size and on presentation measured 6 × 6 cm. The irregular mass was situated in the upper outer quadrant of a large right breast. There was no axillary lymphadenopathy There were no other relevant details. A trucut biopsy was performed which confirmed invasive carcinoma (Fig. 12.1). One week after biopsy, the mass measured 7 × 7 cm indicating further progression, and confirming a rapidly growing tumour.

There are many situations where a breast cancer physician cannot give dogmatic advice either because of lack of evidence, if we are truthful, or because many decisions are personal. A clinician can act as adviser but needs to be sympathetic to the patient's wishes and lifestyle, especially if they are different from one's own opinion. The case described below is an illustration of such a situation.

How would you manage this patient?

In summary, this is a 33-year-old premenopausal patient who had a rapidly growing high grade tumour in the right breast. She had large

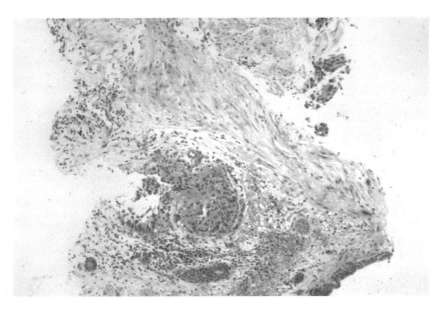

Figure 12.1 Trucut biopsy of breast showing invasive carcinoma (×200).

breasts. Staging investigations were normal. It was decided to treat her with neoadjuvant chemotherapy and she received six courses of FAC chemotherapy (5 fluorouracil, adriamycin and cyclophosphamide). A further but less acceptable option would have been to perform immediate surgery with mastectomy and axillary dissection.

The patient tolerated chemotherapy well and there was good regression of the mass so that by the end of treatment it measured clinically 3 × 3 cm.

What management would you now recommend?

It is more frequent practice to perform mastectomy rather than breast conservation surgery following treatment for a large high-grade tumour. In this case the patient was young and very much wanted breast conservation surgery. This was possible because she had had a good response to chemotherapy and she had large breasts. Wide local excision and axillary dissection were performed. There was a residual 2 cm grade III ductal carcinoma and the margins were clear (Figs. 12.2, 12.3, 12.4). There was no involvement of the axillary nodes and the tumour was receptor negative. She received a routine course of postoperative radiotherapy to the right breast alone with a boost to the site of local excision after completion of whole breast radiotherapy.

On completion of radiotherapy treatment she attended with her husband saying they wanted to start a family.

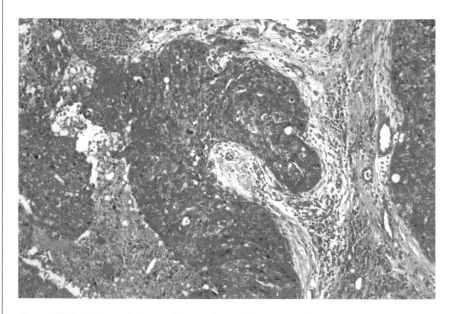

Figure 12.2 Histopathology of breast lump showing grade III invasive ductal carcinoma (H&E stain) (×300).

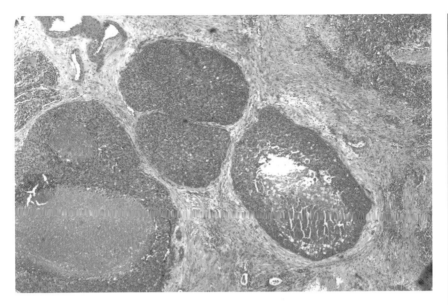

Figure 12.3 Area of high grade ductal carcinoma in situ in lumpectomy specimen.

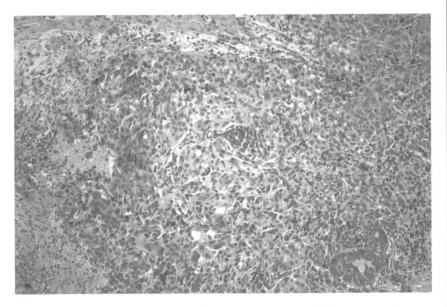

Figure 12.4 Immunohistochemistry showing no nuclear positivity and therefore receptor negative.

What advice would you give them concerning family planning?

As already stated, it is difficult to be dogmatic and this is a very personal decision. However, she has had a serious illness and is at risk of developing metastatic disease. The highest risk period is the early years, and particularly the first two years, and so advice should be given to delay trying to start a family for perhaps between two and five years. There is often a decision to be made about adjuvant tamoxifen, which is usually given for five years. It is undesirable to conceive whilst on tamoxifen and certainly not appropriate to continue with tamoxifen during pregnancy. In this patient's case the tumour was receptor negative and so she was not ever treated with tamoxifen.

What actually transpired, and against medical advice, was the patient conceived two months after completing therapy. The pregnancy went to full term and she delivered a fit and healthy girl. Both remain well over two years later. The only medical history since is that the patient had acute appendicitis one year ago, which was treated surgically and without complications.

What is the effect of chemotherapy on fertility?

What advice would you give the patient?

This will depend on the drugs employed, the intensity of treatment, other additional therapies used such as tamoxifen and, very importantly, the age of the patient. As shown in the above case, there was very minimal change in her periods due to chemotherapy and her fertility was preserved.

Case 13: Acute illness

A 52-year-old patient attended the breast-screening centre for routine mammography. This showed an abnormality lateral to the right nipple indicative of malignancy. She had not noticed any changes in her breast although clinical examination revealed a mass at the site of abnormality on the mammogram. Following confirmation of the diagnosis of malignancy a right mastectomy and axillary dissection were carried out for a 35 mm grade III invasive ductal carcinoma that was receptor negative. There was involvement of seven of the 19 lymph nodes.

Although relatively young the patient has a past medical history of arthritis. She is hypothyroid and is on thyroxine; she has COPD and smokes up to 40 cigarettes a day. She has had a pelvic floor repair.

What would be your standard recommendations for further management in this patient?

This postmenopausal patient presented with aggressive breast cancer; she had a high grade tumour that was quite markedly node positive and receptor negative. It would be appropriate to treat her with adjuvant chemotherapy. She was entered into the Scottish epirubicin CMF trial (the NEAT trial) and planned to give postoperative radiotherapy to the right chest wall and supraclavicular fossa on completion of chemotherapy. She drew the CMF arm of the trial and received seven of the planned eight courses with no side-effects at all apart from fatigue and mild depression. Sixteen days after receiving the seventh course of chemotherapy she was admitted with abdominal pain, slight hypertension and was apyrexial. Clinical examination and particularly abdominal examination was normal. Abdominal X-rays were normal. Her white count was reduced at 0.99 and oxygen saturation in air was 91%.

What is the most likely diagnosis and management that you would recommend?

A diagnosis of neutropenic sepsis was made. She had bacteriological screening including blood cultures taken which subsequently grew *E. coli*. She was immediately commenced on IV broad-spectrum antibiotics but her clinical condition did not improve. Twelve hours later she was transferred to the ICU and commenced on high concentrations of oxygen and large amounts of inotropes. She had a classic haemodynamic picture of sepsis. The following day a laparotomy was performed and an acholuric cholecystitis with ascending cholangitis was found. A cholecystectomy was performed. She was given full postoperative support on intensive care but, after an initial improvement, she deteriorated and died two days later.

Comment

The above case is presented as a reminder that acute illness can occur whilst undergoing adjuvant therapy for breast cancer. The adjuvant therapy may have a deleterious affect and no doubt in this patient contributed to the final outcome. On reviewing the case, correct decisions were made concerning adjuvant therapy. She certainly had high-risk breast cancer where adjuvant chemotherapy is employed. There was a possibility of an anthracycline regime but she drew the CMF arm. The regimen given in this study is IV CMF (cyclophosphamide 750 mg/m^2, methotrexate 50 mg/m^2, and 5 fluorouracil 600 mg/m^2 every 3 weeks). This type of CMF is less toxic than the classical regimen. On the previous six courses of CMF, it did not cause any toxicity and particularly myelosuppression. However, when the patient developed acute cholecystitis two weeks after her seventh course of chemotherapy, she did have leucopenia and septicaemia. It is therefore likely that the adjuvant chemotherapy was contributory to her death. This is a reminder, therefore, that this type of adjuvant treatment can be associated with serious toxicity.

Case 14: Metastatic disease – or not?

A 72-year-old patient underwent a mastectomy and axillary clearance for a carcinoma of the left breast. Pathology revealed a 13 mm grade 2 invasive ductal carcinoma that was receptor positive and node negative. She was commenced on adjuvant tamoxifen but discontinued this medication because of side-effects.

Three years later she complained of pain in her right thigh and buttock which radiated down her right leg and was progressively so severe that it interfered with her sleep. She had no other symptoms. Clinical examination did not reveal any evidence of recurrence of the breast carcinoma. There was no evidence of nerve route compression, no neurological abnormality in the lower limbs and examination showed her hip and knee to be normal. She was not tender over the femur. Plain radiology of the right femur showed a small lytic lesion in the upper shaft (Figure 14.1) and a bone scan showed a solitary 'hot spot' in the same area (Figures 14.2 and 14.3). The radiologist felt these radiological findings were compatible with metastatic disease. The biochemistry profile was normal.

How would you manage this patient?

At times, there is considerable pressure to carry out active treatment and this patient was no exception. The radiologist reported that the patient had metastatic disease and indeed she did have quite marked pain in her right thigh. However, she had had fairly good prognostic disease and a reasonable disease-free interval. Bone scan had only shown a solitary abnormality and this should never be assumed to be metastatic disease without direct evidence. Tumour markers (CEA, ESR, CA15 3) are sometimes helpful. In this case they were normal. A bone biopsy should be considered but would have been difficult to obtain in this case and was probably considered too invasive.

A limited MRI scan of the femoral shaft was performed and showed no abnormality (Figure 14.4). The patient was therefore reassured and given analgesic medication. Over the following months her pain settled. A further approach would be to have repeated the plain radiology and bone scan after an interval of three months.

The patient remains well, in remission and on no adjuvant therapy.

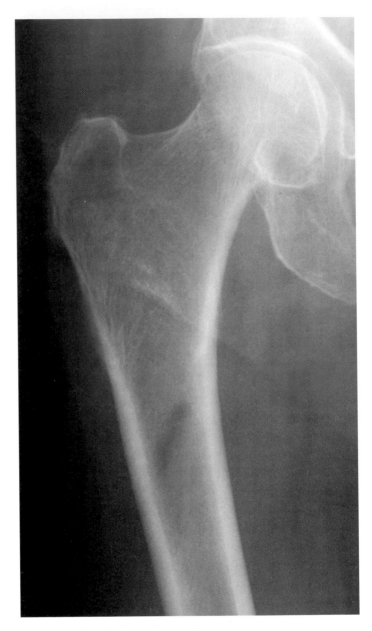

Figure 14.1 X-ray of right hip and upper femur.

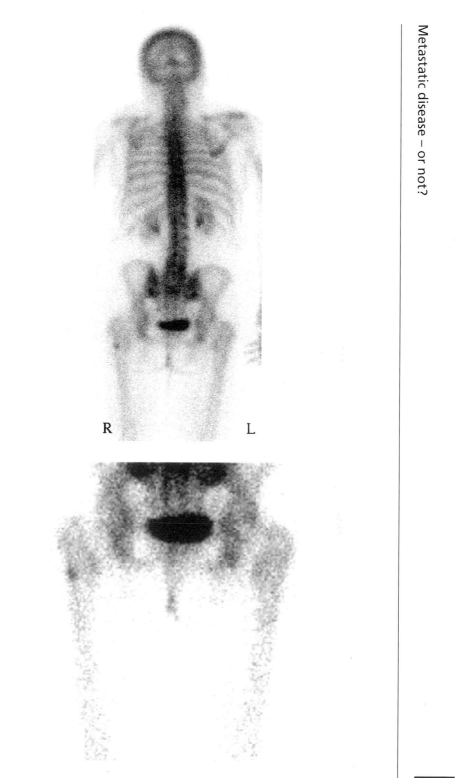

Figures 14.2 and 14.3 Isotope bone scan showing one focus of increased uptake.

R L

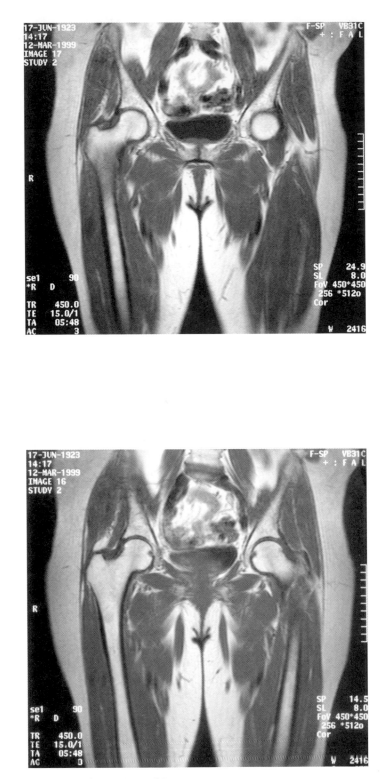

Figure 14.4 Normal MRI scans of femur.

Case 15: The Internet patient

A 36-year-old American lecturer worked in the university as a psychologist. She developed discomfort in the left breast a few months ago and consulted her GP. Ultrasound of a lump in the breast and FNA biopsy revealed benign changes in keeping with a fibro-adenoma. On follow-up she still had a persistent lump and so an excision biopsy was carried out which revealed an 18 mm grade 2 invasive ductal carcinoma. She is single, has no children but wants to maintain her fertility. Her mother had breast cancer five years ago, is well and in remission.

Further wide local excision revealed no residual tumour. One of 22 lymph nodes were involved and the tumour was strongly receptor positive.

What course and management would you recommend?

The plan would be to treat her with adjuvant chemotherapy with either CMF or possibly an anthracycline regime. If she was in North America, no doubt she would be treated with a taxane combination (Taxol or Taxotere) but this drug is not licensed in this country for adjuvant breast cancer. A long discussion concerning egg storage was carried out with the patient. Egg storage is not routinely available in the UK and is not even considered in patients who are under the age of 30. The patient has no partner at present.

The patient did an extensive search on the Internet and, at times, found it difficult to accumulate all the information. Some of the information she had gathered, she found very confusing and this increased her anxiety. She was referred to the clinical psychologist and given a relaxation tape. She also wanted a copy of her notes and this was made available to her.

She was concerned to be treated with CMF chemotherapy if the HER 2 neu status was positive. However, her status was negative and so she agreed to have CMF chemotherapy followed by postoperative radiotherapy to the left breast alone.

After completion of chemotherapy, tamoxifen was prescribed.

Case 16: Breast cancer and pregnancy

A 30-year-old drug representative presented having noticed a lump in the right breast with inversion of her nipple. The breast seemed to become smaller. Mammography showed a suspicious area in the right breast adjacent to the nipple. The diagnosis of breast cancer was confirmed and, as she had a centrally placed tumour and small breasts, a right mastectomy and axillary clearance was carried out. Histology revealed a 15 mm grade 2 invasive ductal carcinoma that was strongly oestrogen receptor (ER) positive. None of the axillary lymph nodes were involved.

The patient attended with her husband and they were very keen to have a family at some time.

What advice and treatment recommendations would you give?

The patient did not have a high risk breast cancer. In summary, she had a T1 N0 carcinoma which was strongly receptor positive. She, of course, was premenopausal. She was advised to start tamoxifen as adjuvant hormonal therapy. The intended duration of treatment is five years. Ideally, therefore, she should be on this treatment for this period of time and then try to start a family. However, tamoxifen was certainly not going to improve her fertility and she may have been unhappy to wait this long. She was given advice about non-hormonal contraception and was also instructed to stop tamoxifen if she did get pregnant as it is contraindicated in pregnancy due to lack of data. She subsequently underwent a TRAM breast reconstruction.

Over three years after diagnosis, she became pregnant and stopped tamoxifen. At 17 weeks pregnant, she developed a lump in the upper outer aspect of her reconstructed breast. This was widely excised without affecting her breast reconstruction. A review of the pathology showed this looked identical to the previous tumour and therefore could be considered as a recurrence rather than a new primary. It was also ER positive.

What further management would you perform?

This is a difficult management problem. The cancer has recurred locally whilst the patient is pregnant and there is a possibility that she has metastatic disease, with micrometastases being more likely than positive staging investigations. In primary operable breast cancer there is no survival advantage to patients in termination of pregnancy. Both the patient and her husband wanted to continue with the pregnancy. Biochemistry profile and liver ultrasound were performed and were normal. Chest X-ray and bone scan were not carried out.

Normally, the patient would be recommended on tamoxifen and given a course of radiotherapy to the reconstructed right breast. Both of these treatment manoeuvres would be inappropriate in pregnancy. Surgical removal of the reconstructed right breast would normally be considered over treatment and inappropriate.

The patient therefore continued with her pregnancy and had an uncomplicated delivery. She breast-fed her baby for three months and then recommenced tamoxifen. It would not be appropriate to give delayed radiotherapy to the reconstructed right breast. Both mother and baby are well and at present there is no evidence of recurrent breast cancer.

Case 17: Resistant inflammatory breast carcinoma

A 39-year-old premenopausal patient presented with gradual swelling and erythema of the right breast over several months. There was no discrete mass. She had a past history of asthma and smoked 20 cigarettes a day. She was married but had no children. Clinically, the appearance was of an inflammatory breast carcinoma; the erythematous changes were mainly confined to the lower half of the right breast. There were multiple, mobile right axillary lymph nodes measuring up to a maximum of 3 cm. A core biopsy was performed which revealed undifferentiated carcinoma and staging investigations were negative (see Figures 17.1 and 17.2). She received three courses of chemotherapy using 5 fluorouracil, epirubicin and cyclophosphamide but after three courses there was rapid progression. There was now erythema of the whole breast and a mass measuring 10×12 cm.

What treatment recommendations would you now make?

The patient had a very aggressive inflammatory breast carcinoma and good combination chemotherapy with an anthracycline had failed. In this situation, it would be very reasonable to use a taxane; taxotere $100mg/m^2$ was prescribed but just after commencing the infusion of drug she developed an anaphylactic reaction with tachycardia, hypertension and wheezing.

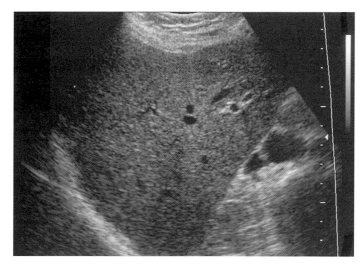

Figure 17.1 Normal liver ultrasound scan.

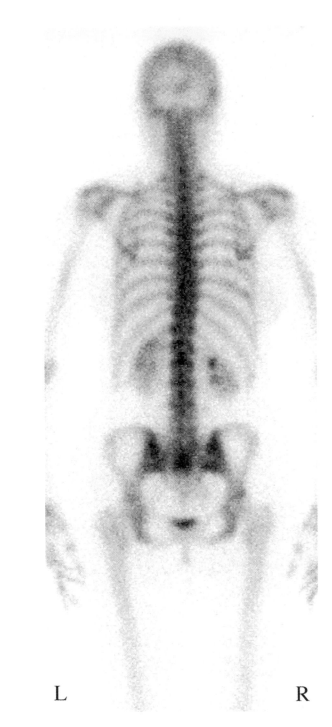

L　　　　　　　　　　　　　　　R

Figure 17.2　Normal bone scan at diagnosis.

How would you now manage this patient?

What further treatment recommendations would you make?

She was treated with oxygen, intravenous hydrocortisone and piriton. It was felt that taxotere was likely to be the most useful drug to try and control her disease and so two further attempts at giving this chemotherapy were carried out with a five to seven day interval on each occasion. However, despite giving a longer duration of premedication with steroids, increasing the infusion time of taxotere and the dilution from one to three hours and giving intravenous hydrocortisone and piriton at the time of infusion, she still developed anaphylactic reactions after receiving just a few milligrams of the drug. She was given salbutamol via a nebuliser. This treatment was therefore abandoned and she was changed to vinorelbine 25-30 mg/m^2 every two weeks. She responded to this drug with resolution of the inflammatory changes of the right breast and a 50% reduction in the mass so that the breast was operable after 10 courses of vinorelbine. A mastectomy and axillary dissection were performed and pathology revealed an 8 cm grade III invasive ductal carcinoma that was receptor negative and involved 17 of 22 lymph nodes.

What treatment would you now employ?

Although the patient eventually had a reasonable response to chemotherapy, there was still bulky high grade residual disease at the time of surgery. There was also extensive axillary node involvement. There was really no further scope for giving chemotherapy at this juncture. She received a course of postoperative radiotherapy to the right mastectomy scar and skin flaps and supraclavicular fossa receiving 45 Gy in 20 fractions using a 3 field megavoltage technique. This treatment was well tolerated.

She was also commenced on tamoxifen although there was little chance of this being effective as she had an ER negative and high grade tumour.

Three months later the patient underwent a laparotomy for an appendicular abscess and made a good recovery. A further three months later she was reviewed in the clinic and was obviously unwell. She had developed left supraclavicular lymphadenopathy and had small nodes in the right supraclavicular fossa, some erythematous changes over the right chest wall which were suspicious of recurrence and hepatomegaly. Investigations confirmed hepatic metastases (Figure 17.3) and bone scan showed a single hot spot in the region of the first lumbar vertebra (Figure 17.4). The therapeutic options were extremely limited but she was commenced on adriamycin 70 mg/m^2 and showed signs of response whilst awaiting HER 2 neu status with the possibility of giving herceptin. She had already received a relatively low dose of epirubicin (50 mg/m^2) in the FEC combination chemotherapy to which she progressed.

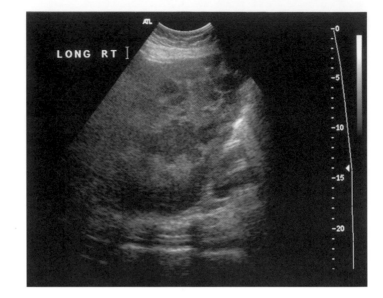

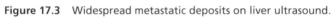

Figure 17.3 Widespread metastatic deposits on liver ultrasound.

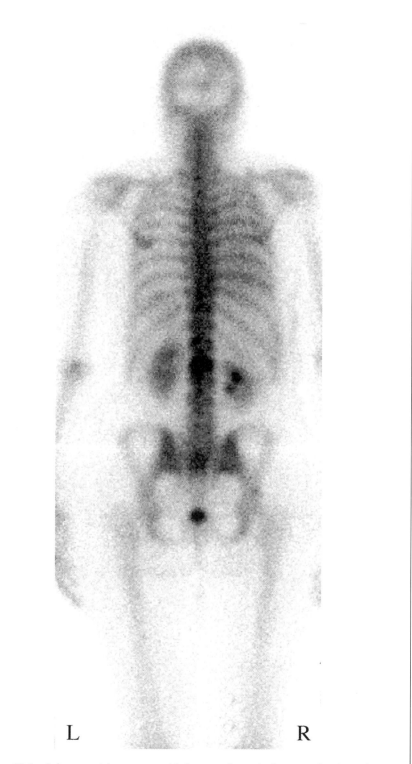

L   R

Figure 17.4 Subsequent bone scan with increased uptake in upper lumbar spine.

Case 18: Axillary lymphadenopathy

A 41-year-old woman presented with right axillary lymphadenopathy. She was well and clinical examination revealed two mobile lymph nodes. There was no other abnormality. She was married with two daughters aged 21 and 15 and had been taking an oral contraceptive pill for 17 years. Fine needle aspiration cytology showed just benign cells but right axillary node biopsy revealed poorly differentiated carcinoma, probably of breast origin.

What management would you recommend?

Mammography revealed that both breasts were dense and there were no suspicious features. MRI of the breast was normal. Staging investigations including full blood count, biochemistry profile, chest X-ray, bone scan and liver ultrasound were all normal.

Right axillary clearance was carried out and the histology revealed five of eight axillary nodes were involved by poorly differentiated carcinoma that was oestrogen receptor negative.

How would you now manage this patient?

It was considered that this patient had a carcinoma of the right breast although the primary had not been detected even by MR scan. The tumour may have been a very small primary in the axillary tail of the breast and removed in the dissection . She received four courses of adriamycin chemotherapy followed by four courses of cyclophosphamide, methotrexate and 5 fluorouracil. On completing this she received radiotherapy to the right breast alone receiving 50 Gy in 25 fractions over 34 days using paired glancing megavoltage fields. No boost was given.

One year later she developed a lump in the right breast clinically measuring 2 cm in the upper outer quadrant.

What management would you recommend?

An excision biopsy was carried out which revealed a grade 3 ductal carcinoma with lymphatic vessel invasion and high grade DCIS of comedo type. The tumour was within 1 mm of the resection margin. Staging investigations were normal. A right mastectomy was then carried out and histology revealed no residual tumour.

Three months later she developed left axillary lymphadenopathy, biopsy confirmed invasive breast cancer and staging investigations again did not reveal any evidence of metastatic disease.

What management would you recommend?

The patient was very alarmed when she again presented with axillary nodes in the contralateral axilla. This could represent a metastasis from the original primary, although it would be an unusual distribution, particularly as it was a solitary site of disease. The patient had no confidence in mammography or MRI of the breast as this had not detected previously any tumour in the right breast. Although perhaps a little unconventional, the patient, husband and clinicians jointly agreed to a left mastectomy and axillary clearance to be performed in case she had a second primary breast cancer. Indeed, prior to the consultation, the patient had decided she wanted a left mastectomy before it was even suggested by the clinicians.

Histology did not reveal any tumour in the breast but 3 of the 11 axillary nodes were involved by poorly differentiated carcinoma.

What management would you now recommend?

Further subsequent management and course

Further chemotherapy was discussed particularly using a taxane but the patient did not want any further chemotherapy at this time. As the tumour was receptor negative there did not seem any indication for hormonal treatment, nor did there seem any indication for postoperative radiotherapy.

However, six months later she developed extensive left chest wall recurrence and supraclavicular lymphadenopathy (see Figures 18.1 and 18.2) which rapidly progressed and ulcerated.

The patient was now willing to accept further chemotherapy and was treated with taxotere intravenously 100 mg/m^2, but failed to respond with very rapid progression of the extensive soft tissue disease and lung infiltration.

She was given symptomatic treatment and supportive care.

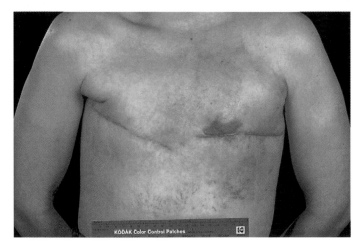

Figure 18.1 Bilateral mastectomy with diffuse soft tissue metastatic disease of the left chest wall.

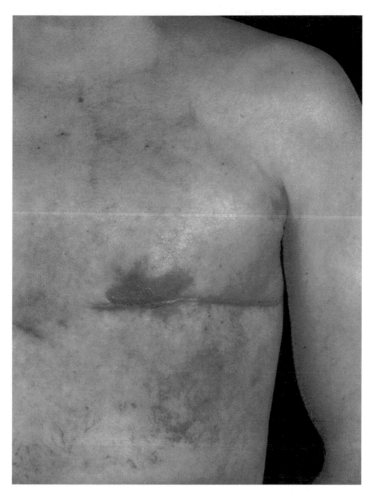

Figure 18.2   Diffuse soft tissue metastatic disease.

Case 19: The unusual tumour

A 42 year-old patient presented with an 18-month history of swelling of the left breast. The size of her breast had doubled over the last two months and caused considerable discomfort and pain.

The patient was distressed and tearful. She had been started on Oramorph. She had a massive tumour of the left breast measuring 26 cm by 21 cm with a purple discolouration and prominent blood vessels over the surface of the breast (see Figs 19.1–19.2).

What is the diagnosis?

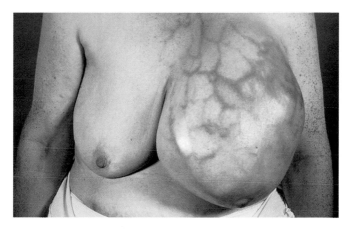

Figure 19.1.

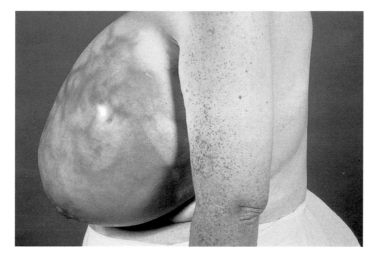

Figures 19.1 and 19.2   Massive swelling of the left breast.

What initial management would you carry out?

The patient had a haemoglobin of 7.9. She was admitted and given a blood transfusion and a trucut biopsy of the left breast showed typical appearances of a malignant phylloides tumour. Over the next two days, she markedly deteriorated and was quite toxic and pyrexial although she was on a broad spectrum antibiotic. She was commenced on diamorphine via a subcutaneous syringe driver to control her pain.

How do you explain her symptoms?

What treatment would you institute?

Radiotherapy to the huge tumour of the left breast did not appear feasible or likely to achieve a response. Technically, it would have been very difficult to administer. Similarly, chemotherapy using possibly an anthracycline combination did not appear to be a feasible alternative. It may have increased the inflammatory reaction of the left breast initially. The patient was already pyrexial and toxic due to the extensive tumour. Urgent surgery with wide and deep excision and reconstruction with a latissimus dorsi myocutaneous pedicle flap was carried out (see Figs 19.3 and 19.4). There had been extensive bleeding in the tumour causing the distension of the breast, and accounting for the toxic condition of the patient and the anaemia. The patient made a very good postoperative recovery. Pathology confirmed the clinical diagnosis of the high grade, malignant, phylloides tumour, the resection margin of which was incomplete at depth and at the superior margin although at surgery there was no macroscopic residual tumour.

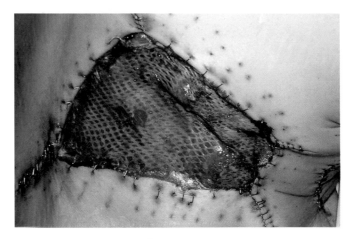

Figure 19.3 Excision of tumour and reconstruction with latissimus dorsi pedicle flap.

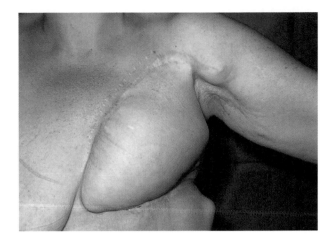

Figures 19.4 Appearance of left chest wall after surgery.

What further management would you suggest?

As the patient made a good postoperative recovery the analgesic medications were soon discontinued. Her clinical condition was now stable so further investigations were carried out including a CT scan of her chest. There was no evidence of metastatic disease including pulmonary metastases. As the resection margins were positive she received a course of postoperative radiotherapy to the left chest wall using large tangential fields and received 60 Gy in 30 fractions using paired megavoltage fields. The treatment was extremely well tolerated and a high dose was therefore achieved to try and prevent local recurrence of this high grade tumour. Adjuvant chemotherapy does not have an established role and was not given.

Further clinical course

Almost three years later she developed brain metastases and after a further remission of a year she died. She never developed local recurrence.

Case 20: The professional sportswoman/Lymphoedema

A 45-year-old squash coach and wife of a GP had a right mastectomy and axillary clearance for a 2 cm grade 1 ductal carcinoma with extensive DCIS. The tumour was receptor positive and was therefore overall, a low risk breast cancer. There was no involvement of the axillary nodes. She did not want any adjuvant treatment and underwent a right breast reconstruction with implant. Three years later she underwent a left mastectomy and TRAM flap reconstruction for a T2 grade 3 ductal carcinoma with involvement of two of eight axillary nodes pathologically from the axillary dissection. She received three of the proposed six courses of CMF chemotherapy but did not want to continue with chemotherapy because of side-effects. Similarly, she stopped tamoxifen after one year because she did not like taking medication and the tamoxifen made her feel slightly sick. However, the left breast carcinoma was receptor negative.

Five years later she developed left supraclavicular lymphadenopathy and was also noted to have lymphoedema of her right arm and a very mild lymphoedema of the left upper limb. Staging investigations did not reveal any definite evidence of more distant metastatic disease. CT scan of the chest confirmed supraclavicular lymphadenopathy with maximum nodes measuring 1.5 cm. There were two or three lesions measuring a maximum of 5 mm in the upper zones which were felt to be vascular or fibrous scars but metastatic pulmonary nodules could not be excluded. FNA of the left supraclavicular lymphadenopathy was carried out and confirmed malignancy.

What management would you recommend?

The patient had developed metastatic disease involving lymph nodes in the left supraclavicular fossa five years after initial management of the left breast carcinoma. It would have been very unlikely to have arisen from her right breast carcinoma. In addition, she had an equivocal but suspicious CT scan of the lung. The CT scan films of the chest should be reviewed.

Radiotherapy to the supraclavicular fossa may exacerbate her lymphoedema and would not be effective or appropriate if she had more distant metastatic disease. The patient was therefore treated with chemotherapy, and received six courses of cyclophosphamide and adriamycin given via a Hickman line because of the bilateral upper limb lymphoedema and lack of venous access. The left supraclavicular lymphadenopathy resolved, there was no change in the lymphoedema, and a subsequent CT scan of her chest was unchanged.

One year later she remains well but had fullness in the left supra-clavicular fossa. She has bilateral mild to moderate lymphoedema of both arms (see Figs 20.1 and 20.2). She has had an episode of septicaemia following infection and cellulitis of her arm.

She is a squash coach and wants to continue teaching, giving exhibitions in schools and travelling throughout the world promoting squash. She is very keen to continue playing. She also wants to continue with household tasks and is a very keen gardener. However, she has had marked lymphoedema especially when there has been associated sepsis.

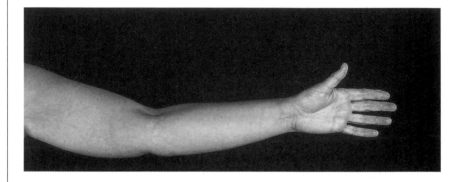

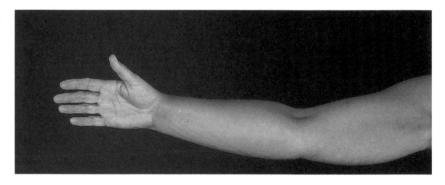

Figures 20.1 (top) and 20.2   Mild bilateral upper limb lymphoedema.

What advice would you recommend?

The patient has used compression sleeves but she finds them cosmetically unacceptable and not that effective. In addition, a compression sleeve has to be worn at least for long periods if not all the time. She therefore doesn't use them. In conjunction with physiotherapy, she has developed her own exercises and spends an hour each morning carrying these out. For household tasks including cooking she uses disposable vinyl gloves. She uses these even for tasks such as making a cake.

She continues to be a keen gardener and always uses gardening gloves. However, most gloves do not prevent all thorns and lacerations. She therefore uses goat skin gloves which are much stronger but more expensive. They can be obtained from some garden centres.

She continues to play and coach squash. In schools and exhibition matches she plays against herself with a racket in each hand. Her lymphoedema is very well controlled providing she carries on with her exercises. On the squash court she always uses a compression glove.

She continues to travel widely but always takes a supply of oral antibiotic (ciproxin) so that any possibility or sign of sepsis can be treated early before a cellulitis or septicaemia occurs.

Further comment

After a good response to chemotherapy it could be debated whether radiotherapy should be given to the site of recurrent disease in the supraclavicular fossa, particularly if it is interpreted that the patient did not have metastatic lung disease. However, radiotherapy to the supraclavicular fossa at this stage would be very unlikely to affect survival at the expense of increasing the degree of lymphoedema of the left upper limb.

Case 21: Late stage disease in pregnancy

A 32-year-old presented with a craggy mass measuring 10 × 15 cm in the right breast and a mass of right axillary lymph nodes were palpable. She felt unwell with mild fatigue, drowsiness and constipation. She was 17 weeks pregnant. She lived with her husband and two sons aged nine and two. She had a previous history of Crohn's disease and had a right hemicolectomy three years ago.

What primary management would you recommend?

She was very unwell and base line investigations revealed she was hypercalcaemic with a corrected serum calcium of 4.94. Renal function was normal apart from a slightly raised urea of 8.1; alkaline phosphatase was 522. The biochemistry profile was otherwise satisfactory. Full blood count indices were within normal limits. A biopsy of the right breast confirmed an infiltrating poorly differentiated ductal carcinoma (grade 3).

What further advice and treatment would you give?

What advice would you give concerning the pregnancy?

Would you carry out radiological investigations?

The hypercalcaemia required immediate treatment and so the patient was given plenty of fluids both orally and intravenously, dairy produce was avoided in her diet and she was given an injection of pamidronate 60 mg intravenously. The management of her pregnancy posed a real problem. It had progressed well into the second trimester and so the risk of fetal complications as a result of chemotherapy or ionising radiation was less than earlier in pregnancy. It would also have been difficult to terminate the pregnancy much later. On the other hand, the patient was very ill with advanced metastatic disease. She had marked hypercalcaemia and it was not clear how this, or its treatment, would have affected the growing foetus. Finally, the prognosis of the patient was very poor and it was even questionable whether she would survive to the end of the pregnancy.

It was therefore decided to carry out termination of pregnancy. This was carried out a week later when she had responded well to medical therapy and was normocalcaemic. In view of this decision, X-rays and bone scan were performed. Chest X-ray showed collapse of T6 vertebra and involvement of T8 vertebra. Bone scan showed widespread metastases involving the skull, ribs, vertebrae and pelvis. Liver ultrasound did not show any hepatic metastases.

Postoperatively, she complained of low back pain with radiation down both legs. Bone scan had already shown increased uptake around the lower lumbar spine and she was tender on palpation in this area.

What further management would you recommend?

She was planned for a course of radiotherapy to the lumbar spine and commenced chemotherapy using cyclophosphamide, methotrexate and 5 fluorouracil. An alternative would have been to use an anthracycline combination regime. Although she remained normocalcaemic, her clinical condition deteriorated and she failed to respond to chemotherapy. She had further sites of pain and palliative radiotherapy was arranged to the left shoulder and thoracic spine; neither treatment was completed, as she became more symptomatic due to recurrent hypercalcaemia and anaemia. She was admitted to hospital for further management and transferred to the hospice four months after presenting with advanced breast cancer. She died six weeks later.

Further comment

Decisions concerning continuation of pregnancy are always difficult but especially when the patient is past the first trimester. This patient already had two children and it was decided that she had a serious medical problem which not only threatened the continuing health of the foetus but her own life. It was therefore decided to terminate the pregnancy. Subsequently, it transpired that she died fairly close to the expected date of delivery if the pregnancy had proceeded to full term. However, in view of the relentless progression of the aggressive carcinoma, it is unlikely that a live and well birth could have been achieved.

Case 22: Hormone sensitive disease

A 50-year-old patient presented 25 years ago with a carcinoma of the right breast and was treated with a right mastectomy for a scirrhous carcinoma. She had no axillary surgery. She received a course of post-operative radiotherapy to the right chest wall, axilla and supra-clavicular fossa. She did not receive any adjuvant systemic treatment.

Four years later she developed a palpable nodule in the right axilla. Staging investigations revealed it was her only site of disease.

What management would you recommend?

She was treated with tamoxifen 20 mg a day and continued on this therapy.

Six years later she developed a soft tissue recurrence again in the right axilla which was biopsied and revealed a nodule of breast carcinoma of infiltrating lobular pattern. Again, there was no evidence of any other disease.

What treatment would you recommend?

She was commenced on second line hormonal treatment with megestrol acetate.

Six years later she developed soft tissue recurrence in the same region.

What treatment would you recommend?

Tamoxifen was reintroduced. With such long response periods she was expected to respond to tamoxifen again although for a shorter period of time.

One year later there was soft tissue progression in the axilla again with small nodules measuring a maximum of 2 cm (Figure 22.1).

What management would you recommend?

She was commenced on an aromatase inhibitor, initially rogletimide and then this was replaced with anastrozole. This controlled her disease for seven years but again there was progression.

What would you recommend?

She was commenced on medroxyprogesterone acetate. The soft tissue disease remains well controlled (Figure 22.2).

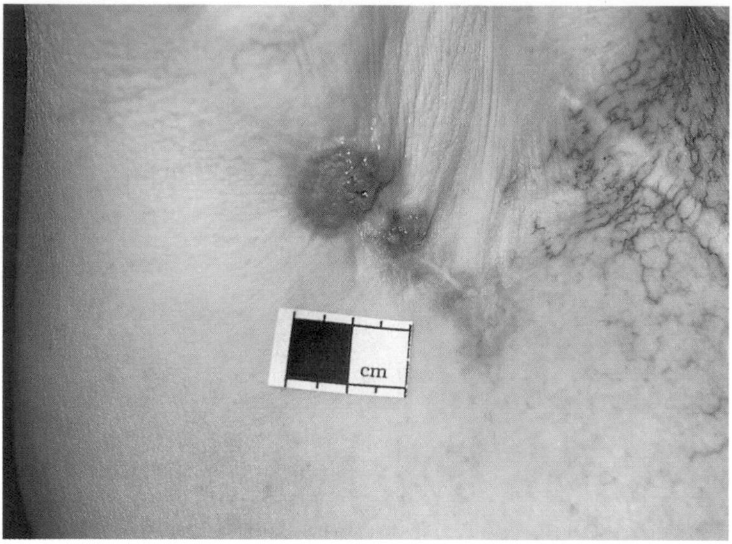

Figure 22.1 Subcutaneous nodules of metastatic breast cancer. Note surgical scars and dense telangiectasis from 'crude' radiotherapy over 30 years ago.

Comment

A further option would have been to excise the soft tissue disease in the axilla. However, this would have been difficult as she had radiation changes extending into her axilla and had had surgery involving biopsy when she initially developed axillary recurrence. Hormone receptor status was not performed 25 years ago but she obviously had hormone sensitive disease.

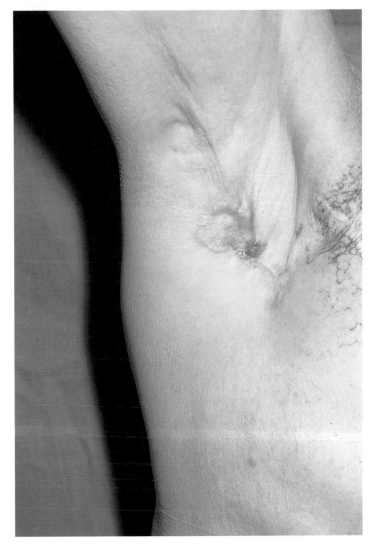

Figure 22.2 Photograph showing regression and control of soft tissue disease after multiple sequential hormone treatments.

Case 23: Receptor negative disease?

A 54-year-old postmenopausal patient presented 17 years ago with a 4 cm mass in the right breast. A mastectomy and axillary sampling were performed and histology reported a 25 mm invasive ductal carcinoma that involved five of the six axillary nodes and was oestrogen receptor negative. Base line tests were unremarkable.

What management would you recommend?

She received adjuvant chemotherapy with cyclophosphamide, methotrexate and 5 fluorouracil given in six courses and then post-operative radiotherapy to the chest wall and nodal areas receiving 45 Gy 20 fractions.

Seven years later she developed right supraclavicular lymph-adenopathy and lymphoedema of the right arm. Further staging investigations were unremarkable. Fine needle aspiration of the right supraclavicular nodes revealed and confirmed metastatic disease.

What management would you recommend?

She was commenced on chemotherapy with adriamycin and received six courses. She also started tamoxifen 20 mg a day.

Two years later she developed soft tissue recurrence on the right chest wall, the largest nodule measuring 2 cm. Staging investigations were normal.

What management would you now recommend?

She was subsequently treated with multiple sequential hormone treatments using megestrol acetate, aromatase inhibitors (rogletimide and then anastrozole), tamoxifen again and then anastrozole again. Each time she responded to treatment.

Comment

She therefore had hormone sensitive disease and must have been receptor positive. Initial receptor measurements were performed bio-chemically and these have now been replaced by immunohistochemistry. Tissue needed to be analysed fresh. If there was a delay then a tumour that may have been receptor positive may have been reported as negative. This obviously could have happened in this patient's case.

Case 24 Solitary bone metastases

A 35-year-old business analyst presented with a lump in the left breast. The diagnosis of malignancy was confirmed and she underwent a simple mastectomy and axillary clearance for a grade 2 invasive ductal carcinoma that measured 3 cm and involved seven of 14 lymph nodes. The tumour was oestrogen receptor positive. Staging investigations did not reveal any evidence of malignancy

What management would you recommend?

Progress

She received adjuvant chemotherapy with four courses of adriamycin followed by four courses of cyclophosphamide, methotrexate and 5

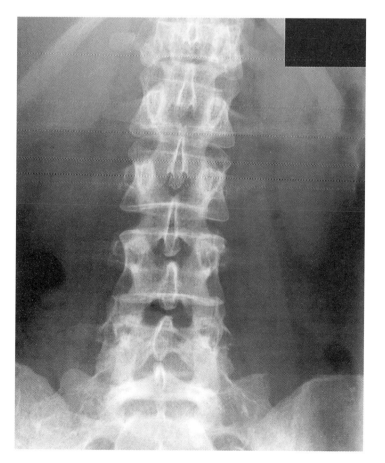

Figure 24.1.

fluorouracil. She then received postoperative radiotherapy to the left chest wall receiving 45 Gy and 20 fractions over 28 days. As she was hormone positive she was recommended to have tamoxifen but this was refused as she wanted to preserve fertility as far as possible. She was also considered for breast reconstruction but this did not go ahead.

Follow-up
Three years later she was well apart from back pain. She had previously been involved in a road traffic accident and had persistent back pain.

What investigations or management would you recommend?

Plain radiology, bone scan and MRI imaging were carried out (see Figs 24.1–24.4). There was partial collapse of the first lumbar vertebra. The bone scan showed two areas of increased uptake and this was supported by the MRI scan which showed metastatic infiltration of

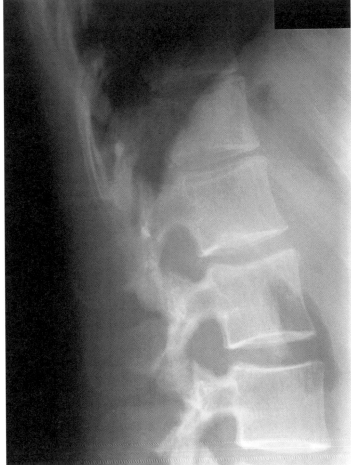

Figures 24.1 (previous page) and 24.2 (above) X-rays of lumbar spine.

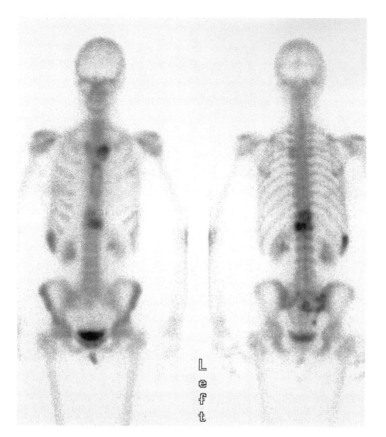

Figure 24.3   Isotope bone scan (anterior and posterior).

the T12 L1 and sacral vertebrae. Other staging investigations were unremarkable.

What management would you recommend?

She was commenced on IV Pamidronate 90 mg monthly for six courses which was then converted to oral Clodronate. She was also prescribed tamoxifen 20 mg a day. After the first course of bisphosphonate, she had complete pain relief and therefore refused radiotherapy to the lower thoracic/upper lumbar spine and sacrum. She has a very active lifestyle, travelling throughout the world for business and leisure, including playing golf and skiing.

Further management and discussion points

- How long should therapy continue with bisphosphonate?
- Should she continue on just tamoxifen?
- What follow-up investigations if any would you recommend?

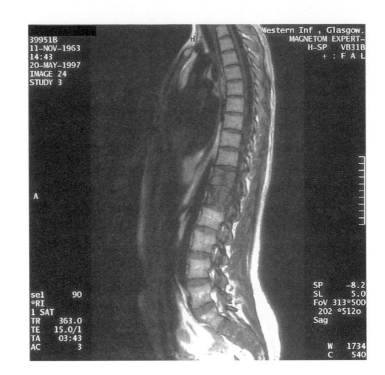

Figure 24.4 MRI scan of the spine.

• What instructions would you give her concerning work and lifestyle and insurance for travelling abroad?

Her company does not know she has metastatic breast carcinoma.

• What recommendations would you give now that she is asking about having a family, three years after the diagnosis of bone metastases.

Further management
She is very reluctant to discontinue Clodronate and so continues on bisphosphonate together with tamoxifen. She has been advised to make sure that she has health insurance when travelling. Further bone scan was performed which showed no increased areas of activity or new areas (Figure 24.5). She has been advised that, as she has metastatic disease, it would be unwise to start a family although it is ultimately her decision.

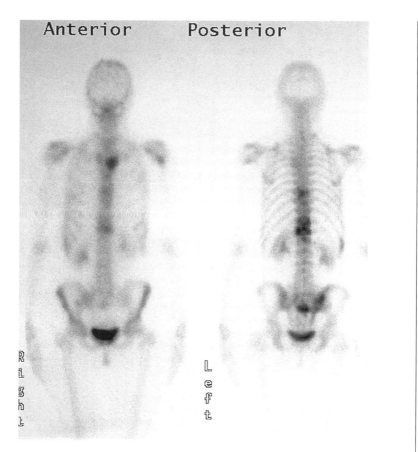

Figure 24.5 Follow up bone scan after one year of tamoxifen and bisphosphonate therapy.

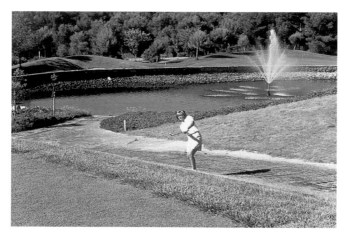

Figure 24.6 Playing golf in Florida.

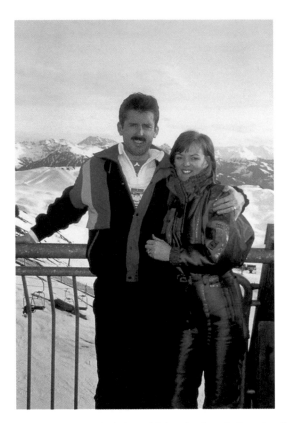

Figure 24.7 Patient on a skiing holiday with her husband after the diagnosis and management of vertebral metastases.

Case 25: The orthopaedic challenge

A 58 year-old secretary in the University presented with a lump in her right breast which she had noticed for two weeks. It was in the lower inner quadrant of the right breast just medial to the nipple. Mammography was suspicious of malignancy and FNA showed malignant cells. Trucut biopsy confirmed the diagnosis.

Mastectomy and axillary clearance were performed and histology reported a 25 mm grade II invasive ductal carcinoma with tumour in the lymphatics of the breast. One of the 16 axillary nodes was involved. The tumour was 100% oestrogen receptor positive.

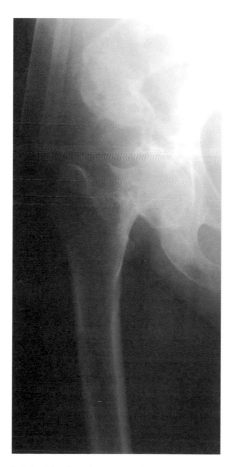

Figure 25.1 X-ray of right hip showing extensive metastatic involvement and a pathological fracture.

What management would you propose?

The patient was commenced on tamoxifen as the tumour was strongly receptor positive. She was randomised in the UK ABC trial and drew the addition of chemotherapy. She had six courses of standard cyclophosphamide, methotrexate and 5 fluorouracil.

Three and a half years later, she developed pain in the right side of the pelvis and X-ray showed destruction of the right ilium, involving the superior acetabular margin. Staging investigations revealed hepatic metastases. However, she did not have severe liver dysfunction.

The tamoxifen was discontinued and she was commenced on adriamycin and received six courses of treatment with an excellent response.

Six months later, she developed pain particularly on walking. There was no history of trauma. She actually felt very well and had not lost weight.

Plain radiology of the pelvis and femur was carried out, together with a bone scan and CT scan of the pelvis (Figs. 25.1, 25.2 and 25.3). Liver function tests were normal.

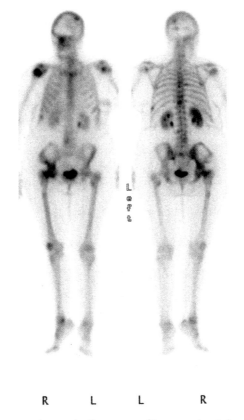

R   L   L   R

Figure 25.2   Bone scan demonstrating areas of increased uptake particularly involving the right hip.

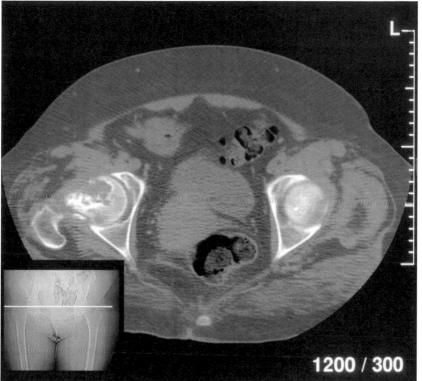

1200 / 300

Figure 25.3 CT scan with metastatic destruction of femur. A large ovarian cyst is also shown.

What management would you propose?

Investigations showed a pathological fracture through the neck of the right femur. In addition, there was a lytic lesion in the upper third of the femur and, finally, extensive destruction of the acetabulum and iliac bone. The extent of disease was clarified with a bone and CT scan.

Ideally, with a pathological fracture the patient needs surgical stabilisation with a total hip replacement. However, this would be unstable with such extensive acetabular and right pelvic disease.

It was therefore decided to give moderate to high dose radiotherapy (40 Gy in 20 fractions) to the right side of the pelvis and upper femur and commence on IV bisphosphonates. It was hoped that this would achieve a good sclerotic response, good pain relief and may enable later surgery. Despite the pathological fracture through the neck of the femur, the patient could walk, limping and with the aid of walking sticks.

At present, the patient continues on this therapy.

Case 26: Aggressive metastatic disease

A 45-year-old patient presented with a previous history of breast abscesses. As a consequence she had nipple inversion, nipple discharge and scarring of the breast. In 1997, she had excision of the nipple and sub areolar tissue. At attendance at the breast clinic, one of the abscesses was again drained and malignant cells detected in the aspirate from the right breast. After aspiration there was a 2 cm poorly defined lump in the inner upper quadrant of the right breast; trucut biopsy confirmed invasive carcinoma. Bilateral mammography just showed changes compatible with scarring from previous sepsis and surgery.

The past medical history included chronic bronchitis, depression, treatment for a psychopathic personality and alcohol abuse resulting in jaundice.

Wide local excision and axillary dissection were carried out and histology revealed a 30 mm grade 3 invasive ductal carcinoma which was receptor negative. As the invasive tumour was 1 mm from the resection margin and there was DCIS in the cavity shaving with lymphatic invasion, she had a right mastectomy which showed no residual tumour. There was no involvement of the 17 axillary nodes examined.

What problems would you foresee and what treatment recommendations would you make?

As may be assumed from the history, this patient had numerous social problems. She continued to smoke heavily despite recurrent chest infections and still drank alcohol. Although she was only 45 and premenopausal she was quite unfit and markedly overweight.

Adjuvant chemotherapy with cyclophosphamide, methotrexate and 5 fluorouracil was recommended as she had high grade disease that was receptor negative. She received six courses without complication. Prior to commencing treatment, liver function tests were normal and chest X-ray did not show any evidence of metastatic disease although she had healed fractures of the left third, fourth, fifth and sixth ribs presumably due to trauma. She was given counselling and saw the clinical psychologist.

Four months after completing adjuvant chemotherapy, she complained of severe lower back pain with radiation down both legs. Plain radiology revealed loss of disc height at the lumbar sacral junction. A bone scan was normal.

What management would you now recommend?

She was referred for physiotherapy and given instructions in using a TENS machine (transcutaneous nerve stimulation). She was given analgesic medication and an MRI scan of the lumbar spine was carried out which showed collapse of fifth lumbar vertebra (Figures 26.1 and 26.2). There was an abnormal signal uptake more suggestive of isolated bone metastases than degenerative disease. Chest X-ray and liver function tests were normal.

How would you manage this situation?

As she had a solitary abnormality she was referred for an orthopaedic opinion. Decompression and stabilisation of the fifth lumbar vertebra was performed with insertion of a bone graft (Figure 26.3). An alternative would have been to give her a course of palliative radiotherapy to the lower lumbar spine. However during her recovery period she complained of pain in the left upper arm and X-ray revealed a pathological fracture through the surgical neck of the humerus with fairly extensive deposits in the upper shaft (Figure 26.4). Technically it was not possible to stabilise this fracture with standard fracture implants. These changes had occurred despite a normal bone scan two months previously inferring very aggressive disease.

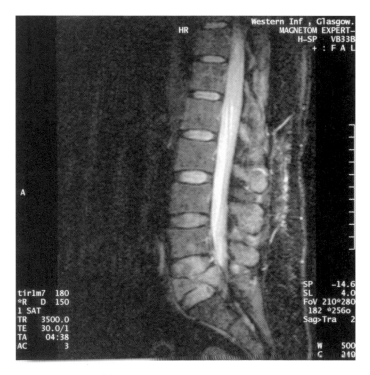

Figure 26.1. MRI scan of the spine.

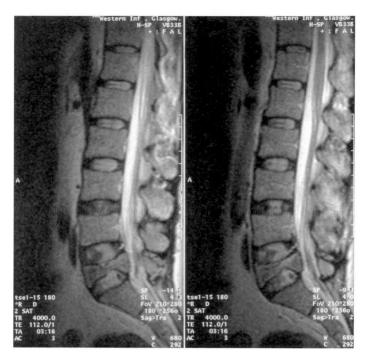

Figures 26.1 (previous page) and 26.2 (above)   MRI scan of the spine.

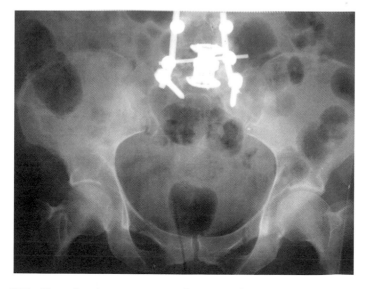

Figure 26.3   X-ray showing appearance after surgical stabilisation.

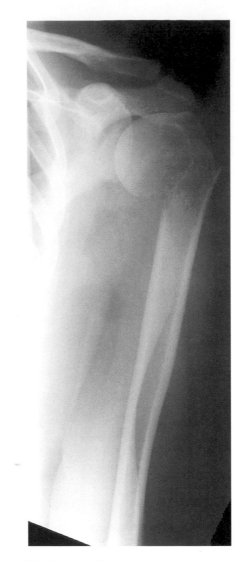

Figure 26.4   X-ray of the left shoulder.

What further management would you recommend?

A hemi-arthroplasty of the left shoulder was carried out (Fig 26.5). Surgery was delayed as the patient was unfit for operation due to a chest infection and she was treated with antibiotics. It was noted that she had pulmonary metastases prior to surgery but as she was unable to use her left arm and in severe pain it was felt that she should still undergo surgery. Liver scan was also performed which showed a few lesions in the liver compatible with liver metastases. Postoperatively she developed bulky right supraclavicular lymphadenopathy.

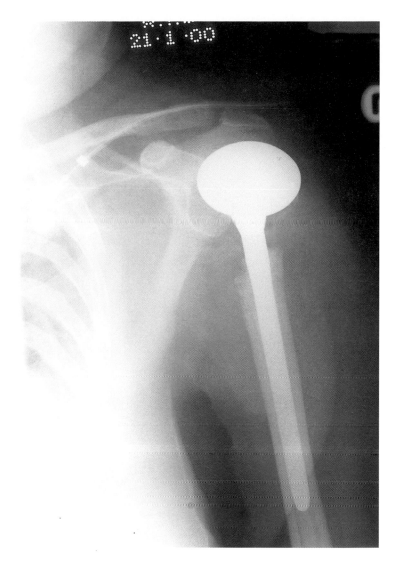

Figure 26.5 Replaced humeral head.

She was not fit for further chemotherapy and a short course of palliative radiotherapy was given to the right supraclavicular fossa and left shoulder following surgery. However, she rapidly deteriorated and became jaundiced due to her metastatic disease.

She was given supportive care and symptom control.

Case 27: Responsive metastatic disease

A 43-year-old investment and mortgage consultant attended having noticed a lump in her right breast adjacent to the nipple. Following abnormal mammogram and ultrasound of the breast, the diagnosis of breast cancer was confirmed and she underwent wide local excision and axillary dissection for a 25 mm grade 2 invasive ductal carcinoma that was oestrogen receptor positive. Three of the 15 axillary nodes were involved. Her husband is a chemist and previously worked with a drug company.

She was treated with adjuvant chemotherapy receiving cyclophosphamide, methotrexate and 5 fluorouracil and received six courses without complication. She also commenced adjuvant tamoxifen as the tumour was receptor positive and received a standard course of radiotherapy to the right breast alone.

Three and a half years later she developed slight breathlessness and intermittent cough. She had no other symptoms and clinical examination was unremarkable. However, chest X-ray and CT scan of the chest showed the presence of bilateral pleural basal infusions and multiple nodules consistent with pleural deposits and mediastinal lymphadenopathy (Figure 27.1). Two hepatic metastases were also detected but liver function tests were normal.

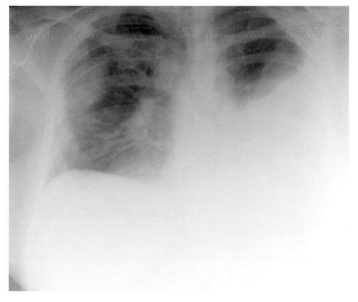

Figures 27.1.

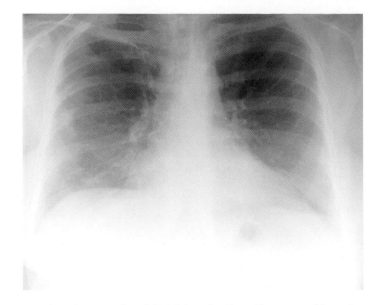

Figures 27.1 (previous page) and 27.2 (above) Chest X-ray pre adriamycin chemotherapy (27.1) and after 8 courses (27.2).

What treatment recommendations would you make?

As she had a long disease-free interval and was hormone receptor positive she was commenced on anastrozole but there was no symptomatic improvement with progression of the pleural effusions which were aspirated. She was therefore commenced on chemotherapy with single agent anthracycline (adriamycin 50mg/m²). This was well tolerated and the dose was escalated to 60 mg/m². She received a total of eight courses with a cumulative dose of 450 mg/m², her symptoms completely resolved. She returned to full time employment and her chest X-ray showed marked improvement (see Figs 27.1 and 27.2). She was able to travel widely on vacation with her husband.

Ten months later she developed respiratory symptoms again and chest X-ray confirmed widespread metastatic lung disease (Figure 27.3).

What treatment would you now recommend?

She had a good response to anthracycline chemotherapy with almost one year off treatment. However, it is not possible or reasonable to continue with anthracycline in view of cardiac toxicity. An option would be to recommence CMF chemotherapy which she received as adjuvant treatment almost five years ago. A further option would be to use a taxane and indeed she received taxotere. There are more side-effects with taxanes than CMF chemotherapy but a higher response rate. She received six courses, again with excellent symptomatic response (Figure 27.4).

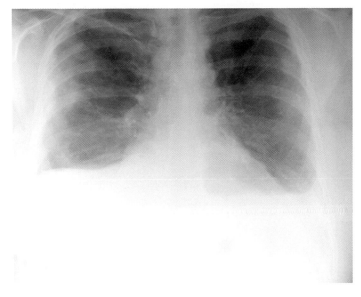

Figure 27.3 Appearance of chest X-ray when symptoms recurred.

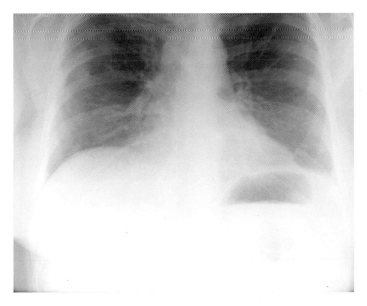

Figure 27.4 Chest X-ray at completion of taxotere chemotherapy.

She returned to full time employment, but returned eight months later with, again, respiratory symptoms due to progressive metastatic disease.

What treatment would you now recommend?

She was treated with Vinorelbine and received eight courses with initially a good response but her disease then progressed on chemotherapy. She was admitted cyanosed and could not talk because of breathlessness. She was commenced on steroids and given continuous oxygen via nasal catheters. She was started on capecitabine chemotherapy which was obtained on a named patient basis. She received 2500 mg bd of capecitabine for 14 days with one week off treatment. She had a remark-able response with tremendous symptomatic improvement and was able to have a holiday in Canada after her second course of capcitabine. After her third she developed a chest infection and became septicaemic and her treatment unfortunately, was unsuccessful. At this time there was no evidence of myelosuppression due to chemotherapy.

Case 28: Unusual sites of metastatic disease (1)

A 51-year-old patient presented with two lumps below the right breast. The lumps were excised and revealed lobular carcinoma. Clinical examination of both breasts were normal apart from thickening in the upper outer quadrant of the left breast.

How would you manage this patient?

Mammography and subsequently MRI scan of both breasts was carried out which did not show any evidence of malignancy. Biopsies of both breasts were performed including the area of thickening in the upper outer quadrant of the left breast and this area alone showed lobular carcinoma. A quadrantectomy and axillary clearance was carried out for multicentric foci of invasive lobular carcinoma with all 23 lymph nodes examined clear of tumour. Left mastectomy was performed which showed a single focus of invasive lobular carcinoma only.

What interpretation do you give to this presentation?

What management would you recommend?

The patient appreciated the rather unusual nature of her initial presentation with nodules in the skin of her upper abdomen. It could be interpreted that the nodule had arisen in ectopic or accessory breast tissue but it is probably more likely that she had a skin metastases at presentation from the lobular carcinoma of the left breast. As the tumour was strongly receptor positive she was commenced on tamoxifen. Further investigations did not reveal any evidence of metastatic disease. However, six months later she developed a small area of induration of the skin 6 cm below the medial end of the mastectomy scar which was very similar to the abnormality at original presentation. It was therefore excised and confirmed recurrent lobular carcinoma. Again further investigations did not reveal any evidence of more widespread metastatic disease and, as she had only been on tamoxifen for a few months, it was continued.

At review nine months later she had evidence of further soft tissue recurrence with subcutaneous nodules over her back. This was the sole site of disease and her hormonal treatment was changed from tamoxifen to anastrozole. A few months later she complained of vague symptoms affecting her right eye. She said that the movement of her right eye was reduced and the appearances were different from that of the left eye. Clinical examination revealed significant restriction of extraocular movements and there was 2 mm of enophthalmos.

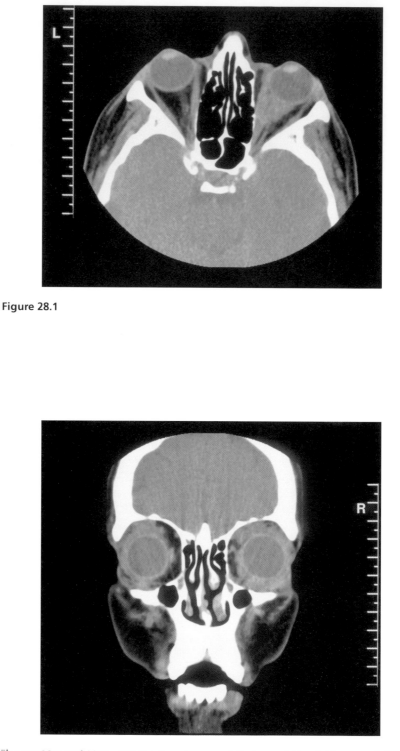

Figure 28.1

Figures 28.1 and 28.2 CT scan showing enophthalmos of the right eye and diffuse changes in the orbital cone.

What diagnosis should be considered?

How should this be treated?

The clinical history and signs are typical of the rare condition of metastatic infiltration of the orbital tissues by breast carcinoma. Classically, it causes enophthalmos rather than exophthalmos.

A CT scan of the orbits confirmed fairly extensive posterior orbital disease (see Figs 28.1 and 28.2).

She received a course of radiotherapy to the right eye using a direct anterior field, giving 20 Gy in 5 fractions. Treatment was well tolerated and resulted in marked symptomatic improvement. Further investigations revealed multiple 'hot spots' on the bone scan indicative of metastatic disease. She was commenced on oral bisphosphonate and following a month of this treatment she said her various aches and pains (which she had not complained about) had completely resolved.

The soft tissue metastatic disease is stable and she therefore continues to take anastrozole. However, it is likely that she will require chemotherapy in the near future. She continues on regular follow-up.

Further comment

The pattern of spread of lobular carcinoma is different from ductal carcinoma. It often spreads to the abdominal cavity with nodules of tumour on the peritoneum and in the mesentery and retroperitoneal disease. There may be associated ascites but it is less likely to involve the liver. In the case described spread involved ocular tissue in addition to skin and bone metastases.

Case 29: Unusual sites of metastatic disease (2)

A 58-year-old patient was treated 20 years ago. At that time she presented with a diffuse mass in the left breast and her nipple was apparently inverted. A left mastectomy and axillary clearance were carried out for an intraduct and invasive carcinoma that involved nine of 11 lymph nodes. No further details were available and receptor status was not identified. At that time, she received a short course of adjuvant CMF chemotherapy followed by a course of radiotherapy to the left chest wall and gland areas. She was treated with a combination of megavoltage and orthovoltage radiotherapy with large fractions per day. One would have expected radiation changes over the treated area.

Twenty years later she presented with multiple cutaneous lesions over her scalp. Biopsy was performed and confirmed recurrent carcinoma of the breast. Chest X-ray and CT scan showed a dense opacity in the left upper zone in conjunction with changes in the upper lobe and pleural thickening at the left apex. It was felt that these changes were compatible with previous tubercular infection rather than metastatic disease. Bone scan showed areas of increased uptake which were interpreted as metastatic disease.

What treatment would you recommend?

With such a long disease-free interval it is likely that she had hormone sensitive disease. She was therefore commenced on tamoxifen but there was soft tissue progression. In addition a chest X-ray showed more peripheral densities and she developed a left lower lobe collapse. She was therefore commenced on chemotherapy with epirubicin (100mg/m^2) and received six courses. She had a good response to treatment with regression of the soft tissue disease. The left lower lobe did not re-expand.

Just under six months later, she complained of deteriorating vision in the left eye and the scalp nodules had progressed and had become painful. Ophthalmic assessment revealed bilateral choroidal deposits, with particularly a deposit inferior to the left disc (see Figs 29.1 and 29.2). Visual acuity was 6 over 24 in the left eye and 6 over 9 in the right eye.

How would you now manage this patient?

She received a course of palliative radiotherapy to both orbits using paired lateral portals and receiving 20 Gy in 5 fractions. Choroidal

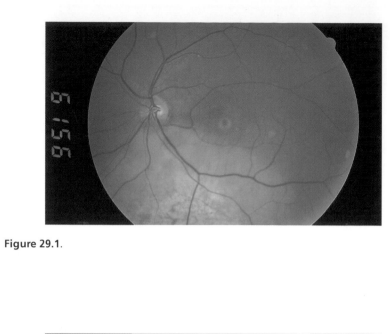

Figure 29.1.

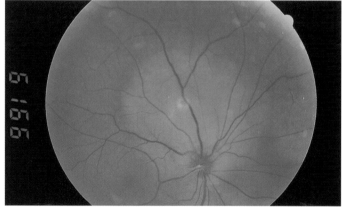

Figures 29.1 and 29.2   Left (29.1) and right (29.2) fundus.

metastases threatening vision are an oncological emergency and require urgent treatment. She had an excellent response to this treatment, with visual acuity improving to 6 over 6 in the left eye and just minimally disturbed vision (Figures 29.3 and 29.4).

She was also commenced on chemotherapy with cyclophosphamide, methotrexate and 5 fluorouracil but after four courses her soft tissue disease was progressing and she developed right supraclavicular lymphadenopathy. The lesions over her scalp were particularly painful requiring opioid analgesia (Figure 29.5).

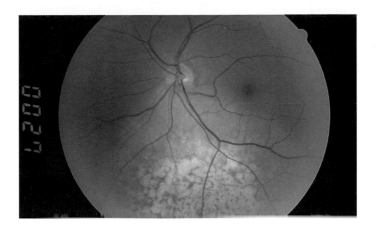

Figure 29.3.

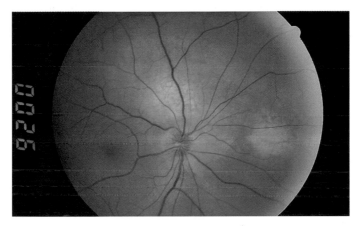

Figures 29.3 and 29.4 Left (29.3) and right (29.4) fundi after radiotherapy showing marked regression of the metastatic deposits.

What treatment recommendations would you now make?

She was commenced on chemotherapy with taxotere 100 mg/m^2 and received six courses at three-weekly intervals. This was very well tolerated apart from causing fatigue and there was almost complete resolution of the subcutaneous deposits over the scalp and marked regression in the supraclavicular lymphadenopathy. Eighteen months later she remains quite well with very slow progression of her soft tissue disease. She has been commenced on second line hormonal treatment with anastrozole. The choroidal metastases remain inactive and she has good vision.

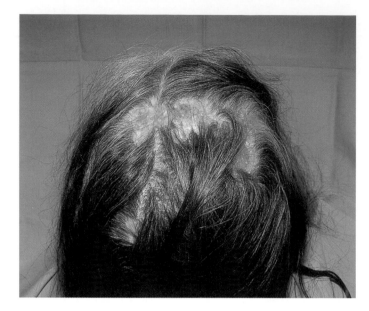

Figure 29.5   Metastatic infiltration of the scalp.

Case 30: The neglected tumour and unconventional management

A 52-year-old woman patient presented with a locally advanced carcinoma of the left breast (see Figs. 30.1 and 30.2). It had been present for at least one year and had gradually progressed. It had caused swelling of her left arm which made playing golf difficult and she therefore sought medical attention. She felt very well. She was still menstruating. On examination she had a locally advanced carcinoma of the left breast, which was fixed to the chest wall, lymphoedema of the left arm and supraclavicular lymphadenopathy. There was a small area of peau d'orange in the right breast with a very poorly defined mass. Trucut biopsy of the left breast confirmed invasive carcinoma. Staging investigations revealed widespread bone metastases (see Fig. 30.3). She was treated with combination chemotherapy using 5 fluorouracil 500 mg/m^2, adriamycin 50 mg/m^2 and cyclophosphamide 500 mg/m^2, receiving a total of eight courses. There was an excellent response to treatment with resolution of the left supraclavicular lymphadenopathy, resolution of the lymphoedema of the left arm, regression of the left breast mass so that it was no longer fixed to the chest wall and complete resolution of the localised changes in the right breast. A further bone scan was therefore arranged to document response and this showed marked improvement with minimal residual increased uptake (See Figure 30.4).

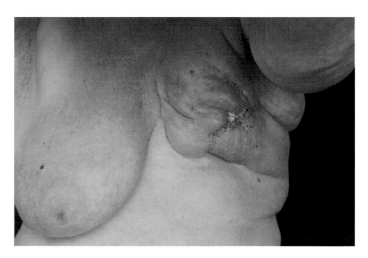

Figure 30.1.

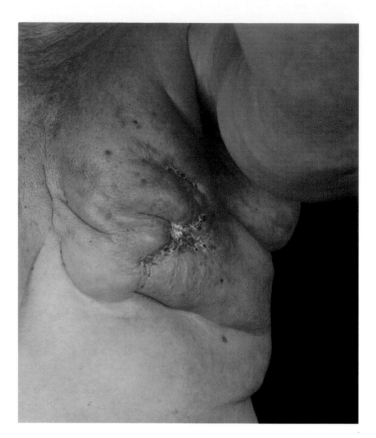

Figures 30.1 and 30.2 Locally advanced neglected left breast carcinoma.

How would you manage this patient?

She presented with locally advanced disease and extensive lymph node involvement. In addition, she had widespread bone metastases and was at high risk of having other metastatic disease, possibly also involving the right breast. However, following chemotherapy, she had such an excellent response to therapy that there was discussion on how to best achieve local control. It was decided to perform a left simple mastectomy despite the presence of metastatic disease. No axillary surgery was performed as it was felt clearance could not be achieved. Histopathology of the mastectomy revealed a residual 15 mm grade 3 invasive ductal carcinoma that was just involving the pectoralis major muscle, a sliver of which was excised with the tumour. The tumour was oestrogen receptor positive. The patient received a course of postoperative radiotherapy to the left mastectomy scar and skin flaps together with the supraclavicular fossa and axilla receiving 45 gray in 20 fractions using a four field megavoltage isocentric technique. At the end of treatment, she developed a skin reaction which gradually settled (see

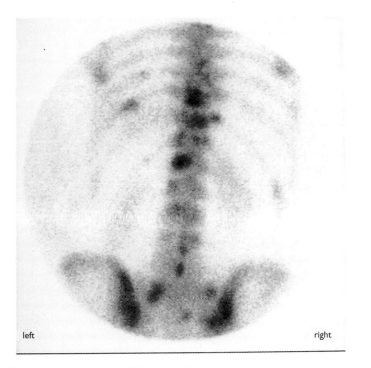

Figure 30.3 Bone scan – magnified view showing central, most active hot spots.

left   right

Figs. 30.5 and 30.6). The tumour was receptor positive and she was commenced on tamoxifen.

She returned to playing golf and having a very active social life. Just under one year later, she developed a large mass involving the right breast consistent with malignancy; there was no evidence of recurrence in the left chest wall or nodal areas. A biopsy was performed which confirmed carcinoma. Restaging investigations revealed some evidence of progression of the bone metastases but she was asymptomatic.

How would you now treat this patient?

A mastectomy and axillary clearance on this occasion, was carried out to try and achieve local control. Histology reported a 15 mm grade 3 invasive ductal carcinoma with, again, involvement of the pectoral muscle. Twenty-one of 24 lymph nodes were involved and the tumour again were strongly receptor positive. A course of postoperative radiotherapy was given to the right mastectomy scar and skin flaps using paired glancing megavoltage fields. Hormonal treatment was changed to anastrozole. Chemotherapy was not given after the second mastectomy as it could not be considered as adjuvant treatment and, although she had

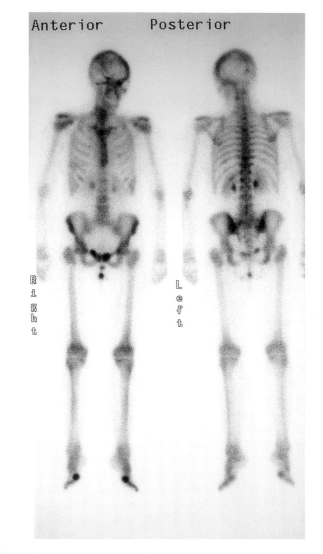

Figure 30.4 Subsequent bone scan showing the whole skeleton.

metastatic disease, she was asymptomatic. The patient remained very well for just over one year with a busy social life and continued to play golf. She was then admitted acutely with marked hypercalcaemia and failed to respond to intravenous fluids and bisphosphonate.

Further comment

Mastectomy is infrequently performed in the presence of widespread metastatic disease. However, it was carried out twice in this patient to try

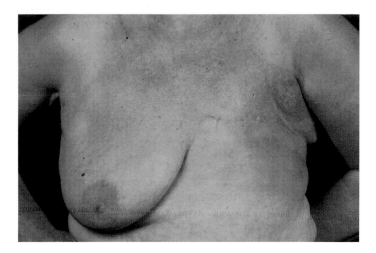

Figure 30.5.

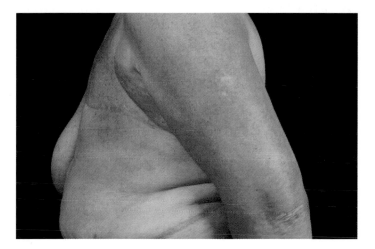

Figures 30.5 and 30.6 Appearance after mastectomy and radiotherapy.

and obtain local control and this was achieved throughout the remaining duration of her illness. This was despite the fact that she presented with an inoperable carcinoma of the left breast. It is quite remarkable that she remained so active and manageed to play golf well right up to her sudden acute terminal illness.

Case 31: Extensive soft tissue disease

This 52-year-old patient initially presented at the age of 36 when right breast conservation surgery followed by postoperative radiotherapy to the right breast was performed for an invasive lobular carcinoma measuring 2 cm. There were no other pathological details and in particular no nodal information. She received 50 Gy in 25 fractions using paired tangential fields followed by an iridium wire implant to the tumour bed.

She remained well and was not on any adjuvant treatment. Eleven years later, she developed erythema and thickening of the skin on her right breast which extended outside the region of high dose radiotherapy given to the right breast. It involved the medial part of the left breast which had become oedematous with peau d'orange and there was a feeling of a dense central mass. Trucut biopsies were performed of both breasts and a small biopsy of involved skin in between the breasts and all were positive for carcinoma. Further investigations did not reveal any evidence of distant metastatic disease.

Before discussing management, the patient said she would not accept chemotherapy.

How would you advise her?

With a long disease-free interval, it was likely that the tumour is receptor positive and would be responsive to hormonal therapy. She was therefore commenced on tamoxifen. On review one month later, there was perhaps some slight regression of her soft tissue disease but it was still very extensive and it was decided to add goserelin as combined hormonal therapy to tamoxifen. She achieved an excellent response with regression of the soft tissue disease and continued on this combined hormonal therapy for five years. However, the disease progressed again and she was commenced on anastrozole, which replaced the tamoxifen, but with no response over the following month (Fig. 31.1).

This patient was still very fearful of chemotherapy. She was head of a Maths department in a secondary school and worked full-time. She was very concerned about her appearance and did not want to lose her hair.

What recommendations would you make?

After very careful counselling she was commenced on low dose CMF chemotherapy (cyclophosphamide 600 mg/m^2, methotrexate 40 mg/m^2

and 5 fluorouracil 600 mg/m^2 intravenously every three weeks). This chemotherapy regime is probably associated with the least side-effects and she was very unlikely to develop alopecia. Indeed this was the case and she received eight courses of treatment with an excellent clinical response (see Fig. 31.2). Three months after completing chemotherapy there was evidence of soft tissue progression again. In view of her concern about the side-effects, she was given oral capecitabine chemotherapy, which was obtained on a named patient basis. She received eight to 10 days of oral treatment every three weeks using 2150 mg bd. The duration of chemotherapy was limited due to mild to moderate hand-foot syndrome. She received eight courses and achieved an excellent regression of her soft tissue disease again.

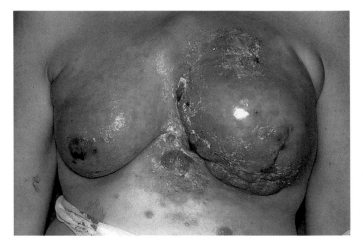

Figure 31.1 Extensive soft tissue disease with ulcerating tumour nodules. Note the swelling caused by internal mammary and infraclavicular lymphadenopathy.

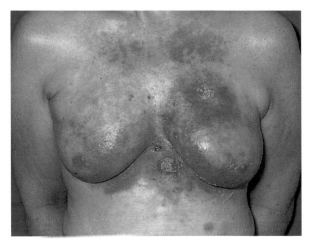

Figure 31.2 Regression of the disease after chemotherapy with CMF.

Six months later she developed further progression of her soft tissue disease and lung involvement. She was then willing to receive anthracycline chemotherapy but failed to respond to treatment.

Further comment

An interpretation of the course of disease is that this patient was originally treated for a lobular carcinoma of the right breast in 1981. In 1992, 11 years later, she developed extensive disease involving both breasts but predominately the main bulk of her disease involved the left breast. She may therefore have developed a second primary lobular carcinoma involving the left breast and spreading across the chest wall. Subsequently, the main site of the soft tissue disease was always the left breast.

Case 32: Male breast cancer

A 70-year-old retired male prison officer presented 11 years ago when a right mastectomy was performed for a 20 mm invasive grade 2 ductal carcinoma. Receptor status was not done at the time but it would be likely that the tumour was oestrogen receptor positive and he was treated with tamoxifen. There was no axillary node involvement. Ten years later he presented with a persistent cough and shortness of breath. He was dyspnoeic at rest. He also complained of sternal swelling which caused some pain.

The rarity of male breast cancer is as well known as is the high incidence of female breast cancer. This, therefore, makes the treatment of male breast cancer both interesting and challenging. Male breast cancer patients tend to be elderly.

Clinical examination revealed that this elderly 80-year-old gentleman had a diffuse poorly defined right parasternal swelling. Respiratory examination revealed widespread rhonchi and crepitations. Chest X-ray showed shadowing particularly in the left mid and lower zones. A CT scan of the chest was performed which showed the large chest wall mass and tumour involving the left hilum (Figs. 32.1 and 32.2). Bronchoscopy was performed which showed narrowing of the left upper lobe and lower lobe bronchi. Biopsies were carried out which revealed poorly differentiated adenocarcinoma.

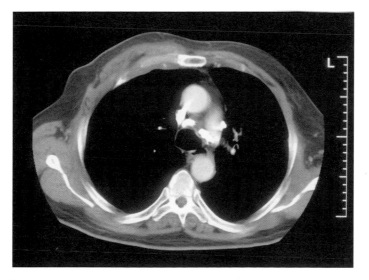

Figure 32.1.

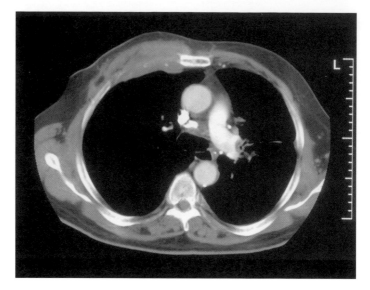

Figures 32.1 (previous page) and 32.2 (above) CT scans at representation.

What comment do you have about this case?

How would you manage him?

There was a long disease-free interval, which strongly supports that this patient had receptor positive disease. Male breast cancer is very frequently hormone receptor positive. The pattern of recurrence would support metastatic disease with the swelling much more likely to represent internal mammary node involvement rather than bone metastases. He also developed lung involvement, which was biopsied bronchoscopically and proved to be adenocarcinoma. It is a possibility that he had a new primary carcinoma of the lung although this would be far less likely.

Since narrowing of the upper and lower bronchi was thought to be causing the dyspnoea and he complained of sternal pain, radiotherapy to the mediastinum using parallel opposed fields and encompassing both sites was carried out. The likelihood of responding to this local treatment was probably superior to any other treatment. In addition the hormonal treatment was changed from tamoxifen to anastrozole. Three months later, although there had been regression of the sternal mass and pain and some initial improvement in the dyspnoea, his symptoms again progressed and clinically breath sounds were reduced in the left mid and lower zones (see Figure 32.3). He was therefore commenced on chemotherapy with adriamycin. He developed quite marked toxicity to this treatment and completed five courses at 50 mg/m^2 at three weekly intervals. He developed mouth ulcers, weakness and weight loss but had an excellent response to the treatment (see Figure 32.4).

Nine months later he remains well.

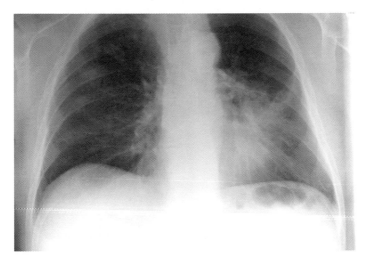

Figure 32.3.

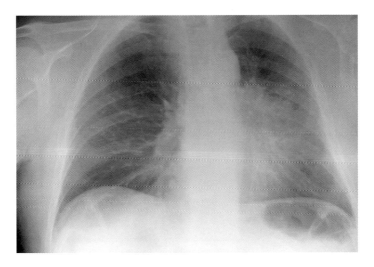

Figures 32.3 and 32.4   Chest X-ray appearance at start (32.3) and completion (32.4) of chemotherapy.

Comment

Chemotherapy was not initially used for treatment of the metastatic disease due to the patient's age and previous response to hormonal treatment. However, he has responded better to chemotherapy than local radiotherapy and second line hormonal treatment but at the expense of increased toxicity. The response to hormonal treatment is slower than with chemotherapy.

Case 33: Spinal cord compression

A 63-year-old patient from a rural village in the Western Isles presented with a neglected carcinoma of the left breast. She had had a lump in the breast for 18 months and it had gradually increased in size. Over the last two months there had been a marked increase in size and ulceration of the tumour which destroyed the nipple. She had a mass of lymph nodes in the axilla. She had lost half a stone in weight.

Clinical examination revealed a fungating tumour of the left breast measuring 12×15 cm with deep fixation to the pectoralis muscle. There was erythema and peau d'orange of the skin.

Further investigations revealed a single lesion in the lung and two hot spots on the bone scan. Biopsy of the left breast revealed poorly differentiated carcinoma.

Discuss her further management

This elderly patient had a locally advanced carcinoma of the breast, which was poorly differentiated. Hormone receptor status had not been performed. Also, further staging investigations were suspicious but not diagnostic of metastatic disease. It was decided to treat her with chemotherapy, giving her cyclophosphamide, methotrexate and 5 fluorouracil. She received six courses of treatment and had a partial response. A mastectomy was then performed and histology revealed a 10 cm grade III invasive ductal carcinoma with involvement of the skin and tumour adherent to the pectoralis muscle. Three of 13 axillary lymph nodes were involved. She received a course of postoperative radiotherapy to the left mastectomy scar and skin flaps, receiving 45 Gy in 20 fractions. She tolerated all this treatment well, which was given to try and achieve local tumour control.

A few months later at a routine clinic review she admitted to discomfort and weakness of the left shoulder and arm, and paraesthesia over C-4, 5, 6 dermatomes. X-rays of the cervical spine and subsequently an MRI scan were performed (Figs. 33.1, 33.2).

How would you treat this patient?

X-rays of the cervical spine showed destruction and collapse of the fifth cervical vertebrae and the MRI scan confirmed this with posterior bulging and spinal cord compression. The other vertebrae were not involved. She was therefore referred for spinal surgery and had stabilisation and bone grafting with a rapid return to full power and

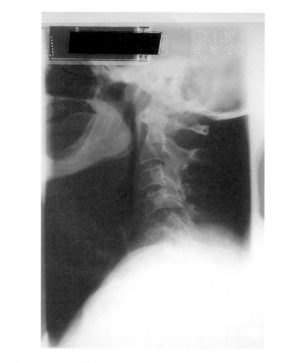

Figure 33.1   Cervical spine X-ray.

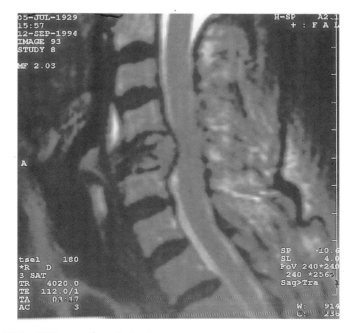

Figure 33.2   MRI scan of cervical spine.

alleviation of the pain and weakness. Treatment was followed by a course of postoperative radiotherapy to the cervical spine giving 20 Gy in five fractions over a week using a direct posterior field.

The patient returned home and was very well. However, six months later she had a severe gastrointestinal haemorrhage and was attended by her GP. She did not wish to be removed from her remote smallholding and died within 24 hours.

Comment

It is sometimes difficult to decide on the appropriate management of spinal cord compression. However, this patient had early neurological symptoms and signs, and a single level of compression. Therefore, it was appropriate to carry out surgical intervention, although she had some reluctance in embarking on this treatment particularly as she was afraid of the city and wanted to get back to her island. However, she was delighted with the symptomatic improvement following surgery and had an excellent quality of life for several months. She did not appear to have active metastatic cancer when she had her sudden, acute, final illness.

Case 34: Recurrent spinal cord compression

A 45-year-old patient presented with rapidly progressive leg weakness and a history of several months of back pain. She had no other symptoms. There was no relevant past medical history. She was unable to walk due to weakness and had Grade 1-2 power in the lower limbs. She had a sensory level at T10. Bladder and bowel function were preserved.

X-rays showed extensive destruction of the T10 vertebrae and bone scan showed widespread hot spots compatible with metastatic disease. There was a thickened area noted in the upper quadrant of the right breast which was biopsied and confirmed infiltration by breast carcinoma. Staging investigations were otherwise normal. Even during these investigations, which were performed very quickly, she completely lost the power in her lower limbs.

What treatment would you recommend?

The patient was treated with high dose steroids and palliative radiotherapy to the lower cervical and upper thoracic spine, and to the mid and lower thoracic spine. She was commenced on tamoxifen. She was transferred to the hospice where she had intensive physiotherapy for six months. Initially she had grade 0 power in all lower limb muscle groups but after two months she could walk with the aid of walking sticks.

Almost three years after her initial presentation she developed severe interscapular pain, leg weakness (lower limb power grade 2-3) and a sensory level at T8. Sphincter function was intact. She was commenced on high dose dexamethasone.

How would you now manage this patient?

The patient received a further course of urgent radiotherapy to the mid thoracic spine with some overlap from the previous irradiation course. She received 20 Gy in five fractions. She was again transferred to the hospice for continuing care and intensive rehabilitation and was able to be discharged walking again one month later. Her hormonal treatment was changed from tamoxifen to megestrol acetate but this was poorly tolerated and discontinued after five months.

Almost two years later she presented with neck pain and difficulty in swallowing. X-rays of her cervical spine showed progressive disease with destruction of the upper cervical spine.

What treatment would you now recommend?

She had a course of radiotherapy to the upper cervical spine receiving 20 Gy in 5 fractions using a direct field. There was no overlap with the previous radiation field. Bisphosphonates were now available and she was given monthly injections of pamidronate infusion for six months and was commenced on anastrozole.

Eighteen months later she complained of increasing pain in her lower back and pelvis and again had signs of spinal cord compression. MRI scan showed collapse of the bodies of T10 and L1 and extensive infiltration of other vertebrae (Figs. 34.1 and 34.2). She received a course of radiotherapy to the upper lumbar spine but did not respond so well on

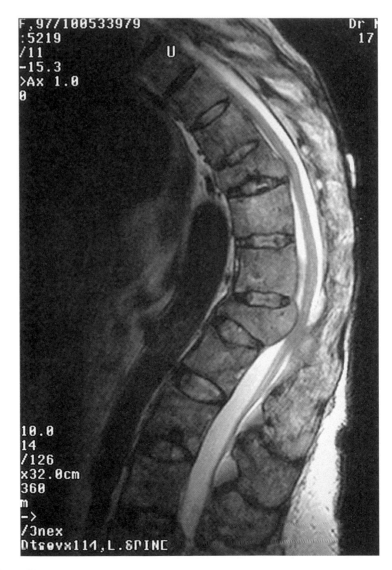

Figure 34.1.

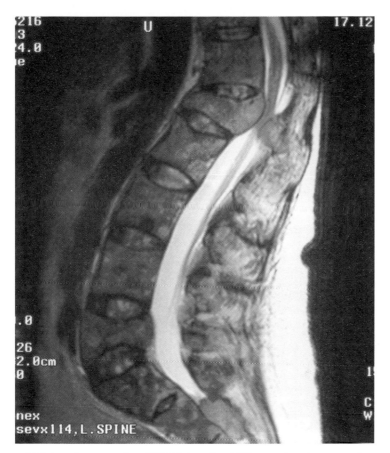

Figures 34.1 (previous page) and 34.2 (above)   MRI scans showing extensive vertebral body involvement with compression of spinal cord and sacral nerve roots.

this occasion and progressed to complete paraplegia with bladder involvement requiring catherisation.

Comment

This patient demonstrates first presentation of breast cancer by metastatic disease causing spinal cord compression. She had very poor neurological function at presentation but made an excellent recovery and survived seven years from diagnosis with several further episodes of spinal cord compression. Breast cancer to bone alone is usually hormone responsive as can be assumed in this case and it is interesting that she never received chemotherapy. MRI imaging was not available during the early years of her disease and neither were bisphosphonates. However, both were used in her management later in the course of her disease. She also demonstrates that re-treatment with radiotherapy can be safely given if it is fractionated. It is also less likely to cause complications the longer the interval is between courses of radiotherapy treatments.

Case 35: Brachial plexopathy (1)

A 57-year-old nursing assistant presented with a lump in the upper outer quadrant of the right breast measuring 4 cm. A mastectomy and axillary clearance were performed for a grade III invasive ductal carcinoma with lymphatic invasion in breast tissue. At surgery there were multiple palpable nodes in the axilla and pathologically eight of 13 nodes were involved. The tumour was receptor positive. She was commenced on adjuvant tamoxifen and given a course of post-operative radiotherapy to the right chest wall alone. She was treated with paired megavoltage fields receiving 40 Gy in 12 fractions.

This patient remained well for five years but then developed lymphoedema of the right upper limb and pain in the right shoulder. Clinical examination was unremarkable apart from confirming moderate lymphoedema. There were marked radiation changes over the chest wall as would be expected. X-rays of her shoulder and bone scan were normal. She was treated with physiotherapy, analgesics and a compression sleeve. She also received treatment with a flowtron pump.

Two years later and seven years after her original presentation, the patient developed rapid and progressive weakness in her right upper limb. She complained of severe pain and on examination there was right supraclavicular lymphadenopathy with moderate lymphoedema of the right upper limb (Figues 35.1 and 35.2). Distally, her power was grade 0

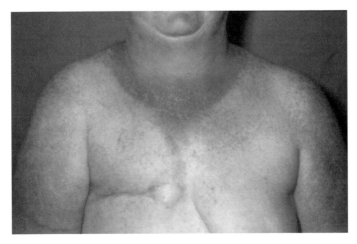

Figure 35.1   Right mastectomy, fullness of right supraclavicular fossa and upper arm oedema.

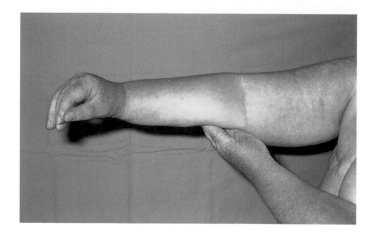

Figure 35.2 Lymphoedema of right arm with left hand supporting paralysed arm.

and she had minimal movement at the elbow. Tone was difficult to assess due to the lymphoedema and reflexes appeared reduced. Sensation was intact.

How would you interpret the above findings?

What management would you propose?

This patient was originally managed seven years ago. One would expect now that a patient with extensive nodal involvement would receive adjuvant chemotherapy. This was not given at the time and it is difficult to say whether it would have made any difference. She certainly did well considering she had a high-grade tumour with extensive lymph node involvement. She was also treated with large fractions of radiotherapy to the right chest wall alone and now oncologists would probably treat the supraclavicular fossa in addition to the chest wall. Large fractions of radiation could have damaged her soft tissues and caused radiation plexopathy. The lymphoedema could have been caused by surgery, radiation treatment or recurrence in the cervical axillary canal or indeed a combination of these factors.

An MRI scan was performed which showed infiltration around the right brachial plexus and supraclavicular fossa. The appearances were of recurrent tumour rather than fibrosis due to previous treatment (see Fig. 35.3). There was also left axillary lymphadenopathy (Figure 35.4). X-rays of the right shoulder showed subluxation of the joint due to paresis by tumour infiltration (see Fig. 35.5).

She was planned for a course of radiotherapy to the right supra-clavicular fossa with careful matching from her previous treatment so that there was not an overlap of radiation fields. She received 45 Gy in 20 fractions using parallel opposed fields. Staging investigations were un remarkable. Her hormonal treatment was changed to megestrol acetate. One month after completion of radiotherapy there was regression of the

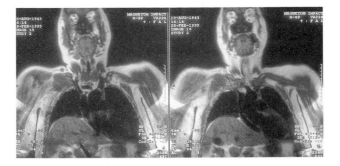

Figure 35.3 MRI scan showing soft tissue recurrence in the cervico axillary canal.

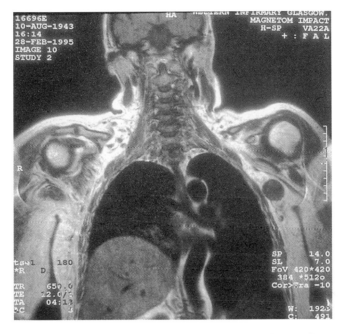

Figure 35.4 Further MRI image showing left axillary lymphadenopathy.

supraclavicular lymphadenopathy, her pain was much improved and power was returning to her upper limb. Orthopaedic advice was sought on management of the subluxation of the right shoulder. She was given physiotherapy and occupational therapy.

Nine months later the patient complained of shortness of breath and had developed a malignant pleural effusion and left axillary lymphadenopathy. The pleural effusion was loculated and aspirated with help of ultrasound guidance. Bleomycin was instilled post aspiration. Further restaging did not reveal any evidence of other metastatic disease. She was commenced on chemotherapy with Cyclophosphamide, methotrexate and 5 fluorouracil. She received six courses and had stable disease whilst on chemotherapy. Shortly after completing

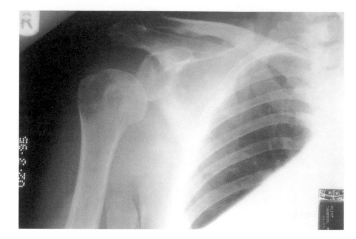

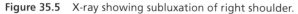

Figure 35.5   X-ray showing subluxation of right shoulder.

chemotherapy she complained of dysphagia and a hoarse voice. CT scan of the chest revealed mediastinal lymphadenopathy in addition to a residual small pleural effusion. After six courses of chemotherapy with taxol and after initial response to the first three courses of chemotherapy there was little change in her disease. Three months after completing this course of chemotherapy she developed superior vena caval obstruction and her clinical condition was very poor. She failed to respond to treatment including a short course of palliative mediastinal radiotherapy.

Case 36: Brachial plexopathy (2)

A 34-year-old premenopausal patient presented having noticed a lump in her left breast in the inframammary region. Clinical examination revealed a 1 cm lump at six o'clock in the left breast and axillary lymphadenopathy. Her mother had had breast cancer in her 40s; she was well and had been treated with tamoxifen.

A mastectomy and axillary dissection were performed for a 20 mm grade III ductal carcinoma involving all 31 axillary lymph nodes. The tumour was 80% ER positive. Staging investigations did not reveal any evidence of metastatic disease. She was considered for the Anglo Celtic trial of high dose chemotherapy but refused to enter and so she received the conventional arm of treatment with four courses of epirubicin followed by eight courses of CMF chemotherapy. Two months prior to completing chemotherapy she complained of pain down the outer aspect of her left arm and there was reduced pinprick sensation over C5 and 6 dermatomes. X-rays of the cervical spine revealed loss of disc space between C5 and 6 vertebrae and she was initially diagnosed as having cervical root compression and given a neck brace and analgesic medication. Her symptoms did not settle and so she immediately went on to have an MRI scan which showed increased signal, with nodularity in association with the axillary vessels suggestive of malignant infiltration (Fig. 36.1).

How would you manage this patient?

This young woman presented with an aggressive carcinoma of the breast with extensive lymph node involvement indicative of a poor prognosis. She relapsed whilst completing extended conventional chemotherapy

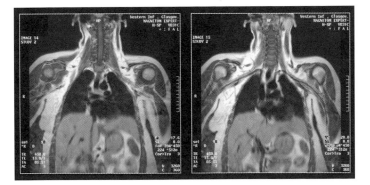

Figure 36.1 MRI scan just after completing adjuvant treatment.

which infers a very poor prognosis. However, staging investigations did not reveal any evidence of lung, liver or bone metastases. She was commenced on analgesic medication including MST and given a course of radiotherapy to the left supraclavicular fossa and axilla and the cervicoaxillary canal and received 45 Gy in 20 fractions using a direct anterior field with a postaxillary field to increase the midline dose in the axillary. By the end of her course of radiotherapy she felt better and was able to reduce the dose of MST. However, almost nine months later, she complained of further pain radiating down her left arm and further MRI scans showed soft tissue changes surrounding the left brachial plexus which were interpreted as fibrosis. There was no progression of the appearances on MRI scan (Fig. 36.2).

Whilst on regular review and many months after recurrence from the cervicoaxillary canal she developed rapidly progressive paresis of the left upper limb and muscle wasting. She had grade 0 power. A further MRI scan revealed changes suggestive of recurrence rather than fibrosis at this stage (Fig. 36.3). Staging investigations again were unremarkable.

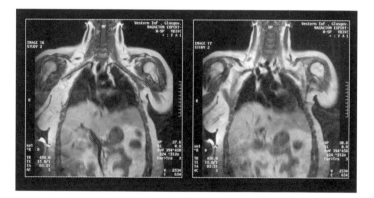

Figure 36.2   Follow up MRI scan.

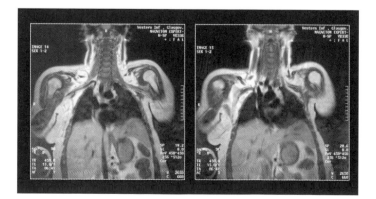

Figure 36.3   MRI scan at time of paresis of left upper limb.

How would you now manage this patient?

This patient has persistent regional disease, which has recurred after radiotherapy and proved resistant to chemotherapy. It is not possible to give further radiotherapy and probably would not be helpful anyway. Her pain was controlled on a cocktail of drugs including gabapentin, S Ketamine (which is given orally), hydromorphone and amitriptyline. She was commenced on chemotherapy with vinorelbine 30 mg/m^2 two weekly and by the third course of treatment her pain had completely resolved and her analgesic medication was reduced. She still has no power in the left upper limb and her arm is supported in a collar and cuff with a sling.

Case 37: Brain metastases

A 38-year-old premenopausal patient presented with a small lump in the left breast. A diagnosis of breast cancer was confirmed and she underwent left breast conservation surgery and axillary dissection for a 25 mm grade III invasive ductal carcinoma with lymphatic invasion. There was DCIS and invasive tumour around the margins of excision. The invasive tumour was 60% ER positive. Two of the 11 axillary nodes were involved. A mastectomy was carried out which revealed residual invasive tumour and DCIS around the nipple. Postoperatively she received six courses of adjuvant chemotherapy with cyclophosphamide, methotrexate and 5 fluorouracil and was commenced on tamoxifen but discontinued this herself after three years because of vaginal bleeding. She also underwent breast reconstruction and then failed to attend follow-up clinics.

She was referred back four years after her original presentation with several subcutaneous lumps around the reconstructed left breast. She also complained of a dry unproductive cough and respiratory examination revealed that she had a few rhonchi only. One nodule was excised which confirmed recurrent breast carcinoma. Chest X-ray was suspicious and CT scan confirmed several very small lung metastases (Figures 37.1 and 37.2).

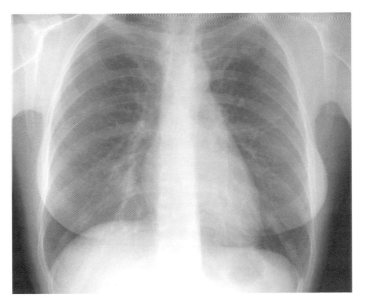

Figure 37.1.

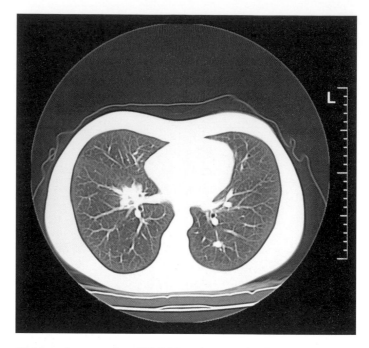

Figures 37.1 (previous page) and 37.2 (above) Investigations at time of presentation of respiratory symptoms.

How would you manage this patient?

The patient was commenced on tamoxifen and responded. There was improvement in her respiratory symptoms, and resolution of the two remaining subcutaneous nodules. It would have also been appropriate to give her further chemotherapy but her tumour was hormone sensitive and she had a reasonable chance of responding to less toxic hormonal treatment.

One year later, she complained of frontal headaches. She had no other symptoms and clinical examination was satisfactory with no neurological signs. Brain scan showed multiple metastases (Fig. 37.3). There was no evidence of progression of her soft tissue or metastatic lung disease (see Figure 37.4).

How would you manage this patient?

She was commenced on steroids and given a course of radiotherapy to the whole brain receiving 20 Gy in five fractions using paired lateral portals. She was unable to tail off her steroids quickly due to recurrent headaches. Six months later she was off steroids and working full time.

However, a further six months later whilst on holiday in France she suddenly became ill, had severe headache and was confused. A CT brain scan showed recurrent tumour, particularly in the posterior fossa (Fig. 37.5). She also had triventricular hydrocephaly.

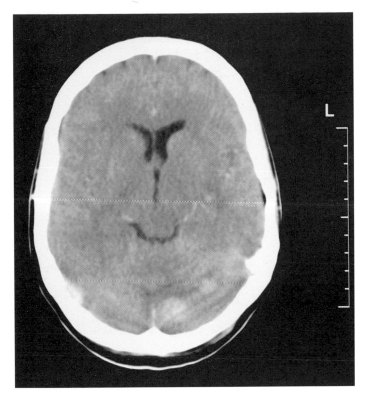

Figure 37.3   CT brain scan at time of headaches.

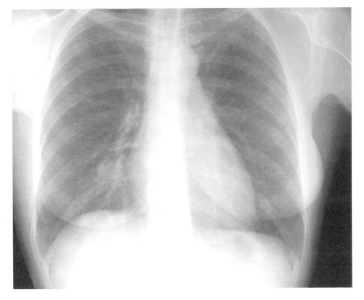

Figure 37.4   Chest X-ray showing stable metastatic lung disease.

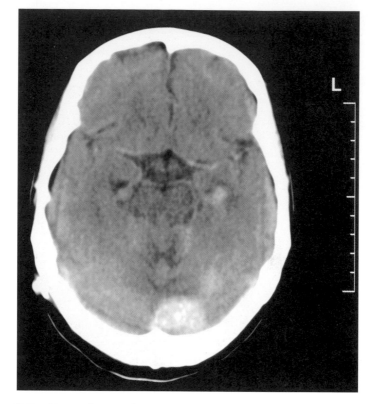

Figure 37.5 CT scan showing further brain metastases.

How would you now manage this patient?

An intraventricular shunt was inserted and she was commenced on steroids again (Figure 37.6). It would be possible although not ideal to give her a further course of radiotherapy as she had had a reasonable response to her first course over a year ago. Chemotherapy is not usually given in this situation because the drugs normally employed do not cross the blood–brain barrier. However, the blood–brain barrier may well be disrupted due to metastatic disease and also to the treatment that she had already received. Responses have been seen in similar situations.

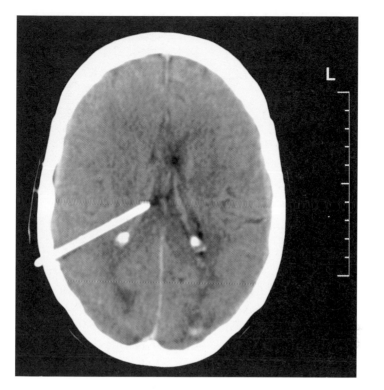

L

Figure 37.6 Interventricular shunt positioned in ventricle.

Appendix I

Trial name and date	Organisation	Address
ABC (pre/post) (Closed Oct 2000)	UKCCCR	ABC Trials Office CTSU 15 Cotswold Rd Sutton Surrey SM2 5 NG
ABO 1	UKCCCR	MRC Clinical Trials Unit Cancer Division 222 Euston Rd London NW1 2DA
Anglo Celtic 1 & 2 1=closed June 1999	Anglo Celtic Cooperative Oncology Group	Scottish Cancer Therapy Network Trinity Park House South Trinity Rd Edinburgh EH5 35Q
ATAC (Closed March 1999)	AstraZeneca & Cancer Research Campaign (CRC) Breast Cancer Trials Group	CRC Trials Data Centre 10 Cambridge Terrace London NW1 4J
ATTOM	UKCCCR	CRC Institute for Cancer Studies The Medical School University of Birmingham Edgbaston Birmingham B15 2TA
Epi/CMF (Neat) (closed April 2001)	CRC	Scottish Cancer Therapy Network Trinity Park House South Trinity Rd Edinburgh EH5 3SQ Or The NEAT Trials Office CRC Institute of Cancer Studies University of Birmingham Edgbaston Birmingham B15 2TT

SECRAB	CRC	Clinical Trials Unit CRC Institute of Cancer Studies University of Birmingham Edgbaston Birmingham B15 2TT
UK DCIS (closed Oct 1998)	UKCCCR	UKCCCR PO Box 123 Lincoln's Inn Field London WC 2A 3PX
START	UKCCCR	Clinical Trials & Statistics Unit Section of Epidemiology The Institute of Cancer Research Block D 15 Cotswold Rd Sutton Surrey SM2 5NG
EORTC Trial D (closed May 1999)	EORTC	EORTC Data Centre Avenue E Mounier 83 bte 11 B-1200 Brussels Belgium
TACT	UKCCCR	TACT Trials Office CTSU Section of Epidemiology The Institute of Cancer Research Block D 15 Cotswold Rd Sutton Surrey SM2 5NG
BASO 2 (closed Oct 2000)	UKCCCR	Professional Unit of Surgery City Hospital Nottingham NG5 1PB

Appendix II

Chemotherapy drugs

Anthracycline
  Adriamycin
  Epirubicin
Bleomycin
Capecitabine
Cyclophosphamide
Methotrexate
5-Fluorouracil
Melphalan
Mesna
Pamidronate infusion
Taxane:-
  Taxol
  Taxotere
Thiotepa
Vinorelbine

Appendix III

Hormonal therapy

Anastrozole
Megestrol Acetate
Medroxyprogesterone Acetate
Rogletimide
Tamoxifen
Goserelin

Appendix IV

Other drugs

Amitriptyline
Bisphosphonates
Clodronate
Dexamethasone
Diamorphine
Gabapentin
Herceptin
Hydromorphone
Inotropes
M.S.T.
Oramorph
Pamidronate
Piritron
S. Ketamine
Steroids

Appendix V

Recommended reading list

1. Early Breast Cancer Trialists' Collaborative Group. Ovarian ablation in early breast cancer: overview of the randomised trials. *Lancet* 1996; **348**: 1189-96.

2. Early Breast Cancer Trialists' Collaborative Group. Tamoxifen for early breast cancer: an overview of the randomised trials. *Lancet* 1999; **351**: 1451-67.

3. Early Breast Cancer Trialists' Collaborative Group. Polychemotherapy for early breast cancer: an overview of the randomised trials. *Lancet* 1998; **352**: 930-42.

4. Harris, Lippman, Moyrow, Osbourne. Lippincott. Diseases of the Breast; Lippincott Williams & Wilkins 2000.

5. Klijin JGM, Blamey RW, Boccardo F, Tominaga T et al. Combined tamoxifen and luteinuzing hormone-releasing hormone (LHRH) agonist versus LHRH agonist alone in premenopausal advanced breast cancer: A meta-analysi of four randomised trials. *Journal of Clinical Oncology* 2001; **19**(2): 343-353.

6. Morgan M, Warren R, Querci delta Rovere G. Early Breast Cancer – from screening to multi disciplinary management; Harwood academic 1998.

7. Hayes DF. Breast Cancer. Skarin AT (ed) Atlas of Diagnostic Oncology 2nd Edition. Chapter 8; 1996.

8. Kaufmann M. Luteinizing hormone-releasing hormone analogues in early breast cancer: Updated status on ongoing clinical trials. *British Journal of Cancer* 1998. **78**(suppl 4): 9-11

Index